The Curve of the World tells the story of the author's relationship with a remarkable spiritual teacher, while drawing connections between spirituality and social justice, music and devotion. As the author eventually faces serious illness, he comes to explore the link between body, mind, and spirit. This is a circular journey toward understanding through the spiritual heart of yoga.

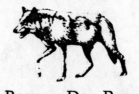

BOTTOM DOG PRESS

THE CURVE OF THE WORLD

INTO THE SPIRITUAL HEART OF YOGA

A MEMOIR

Andy Douglas

"…and the end of all our exploring will be to arrive
where we started and know the place for the first time."
—T. S. Eliot

MEMOIR SERIES
BOTTOM DOG PRESS
HURON, OHIO

Bottom Dog Press
PO Box 425/ Huron, OH 44839
http://smithdocs.net
Lsmithdog@aol.com
Credits
General Editor: Larry Smith
Associate Editor: Laura Smith
Cover Design: Susanna Sharp-Schwacke

Dedication

Anandamurti, for his love and inspiration.

Lois, for her love and companionship.

My family, for their love and support.

Acknowledgments

This is a personal story, and I worked hard to find the emotional truth within it. But it's also a work of creative nonfiction, and in order to create a narrative flow I sometimes relied on nonfiction techniques such as compression of time, conflation of place, and re-creation of dialogue. In one instance, a composite character was created out of two people. It is also, in part, the story of a spiritual organization, yet it is not an official representation of that organization. If I have left out any important aspects relating to this spiritual path, I take responsibility for all such omissions or errors.

There are many people who helped me along the way. Thank you to Patricia Foster and Marilyn Abildskov, who read and encouraged my early drafts. Thanks to other NWP professors Robin Hemley, Susan Lohafer, and Paul Diehl. Tim Bascom, Eric Jones and Kaoverii Weber gave helpful feedback on later drafts. I'm grateful for the support and help of the Travelers Writing Group: Tim and Eric, Lois Cole, Cecile Goding and Amy Kolen. I thank former Travelers Faith Adiele and Judy Copeland. A fellowship at Vermont Studio Center, as well as residencies at Kimmel Harding Nelson Center and the Prairie Center of the Arts allowed me time to work on the manuscript. Thanks to Larry Smith at Bottom Dog for his excellent suggestions. To Ansen Seale for advice on the cover and for taking the author photo. And to Dada Vedaprajinananda for designing my website, www.andydouglas.net.

PROLOGUE

November 23rd, 2004. Stars streaming bright, our plane descended through the atmosphere, down toward clouds in the moonlight resembling rugged white mountains. After a few minutes of wispy obscurity, we popped through to a new layer of sky above the Indian subcontinent. As the view cleared, I peered past the wing; far below I could see the lights of the great city of Bombay sparkling like a necklace, a vast luminous grid girded by the dark curve of the Arabian Sea. Banking over the bay, guided by the rotating red beacons of the airport runway, we made our approach.

Upon landing, I fumbled for my overhead luggage, bumping sheepishly into the other passengers as we moved down the accordion gangplank. It had been a long flight from Chicago, and I was tired, too, from weeks of intensive preparation for this trip. Tired, but happy. Soon, I thought, tomorrow or the next day, I would board a train for the long journey across India to Calcutta.

Inside the terminal I followed the crowd as it shuffled its way back and forth behind cordon ropes. Indians, Eastern Europeans, Arabs, a few Westerners, united in our sleeplessness, all inched along in the immigration line, yawning and glancing curiously at each other.

An Indian man in front of me turned and smiled. Something in the cast of his cheeks reminded me of another smile I knew very well. And in a moment, my mind somersaulted away from this stuffy entrance hall in the Bombay International Airport, vaulted easily over the previous twenty years, and landed in a lush garden outside a house in southern Calcutta. It all came back: my *guru* singing a devotional song he'd just composed, his voice warbling out over the green space. Clean-shaven, immaculately dressed, with thinning black hair and black-framed eyeglasses, this man's radiant smile sparkled beneath eyes full of joy.

By the time of his death in 1990, Prabhat Ranjan Sarkar had composed over 5000 songs. They were starkly beautiful compositions expressing the mystic's desire for God, songs that lit me up like a sparkler when I heard or sang them. This music was the main reason I'd come back to India, a soundtrack to my journey, a phonograph needle set down into the grooves of my time here.

In Calcutta I would study the Bengali language and help to translate some of these songs into English. A grant from a midwestern university was financing the trip. But this was not an academic junket.

You came into my heart and awakened me from dull slumber,
I was tired from my journey; You painted my mind with your
bright hue.

Humming to myself, I stepped forward, finally, to the immigration counter, where something unexpected happened. A bald man in a white uniform with epaulets on the shoulders glanced at my passport and typed a few keystrokes into his computer. He looked up at my face, and back at the computer screen.

He looked up. He looked down. Then, with a strange smile, he asked me to proceed to a nearby room and wait.

The needle skipped. And my heart plummeted.

Not exactly sure what was going on, but with a faint suspicion, I plopped onto a hard plastic chair in the dingy immigration office. A series of low-level bureaucrats scuttled in and out of the room. I pleaded with one of them.

"I'm here as a student. Can't you tell me what's going on?" No one spoke to me. I simply didn't exist.

An elderly European man sitting across from me had managed to come to India without a visa, and I watched as an airline official went to bat for him with the immigration chief. The airline man knew he had to be obsequious. "Please, sir. I would not ask, but it is only that he is a very old man. Isn't there something you could do? Please, sir?"

The boss shook his head. "There is nothing I can do."

The city of Bombay with all its bustling activity beckoned only a few yards beyond a large glass window. Officials busied themselves— *click click click*—with the typing of reports on manual typewriters, and continued to ignore me. The crowd in the hall thinned out, then emptied, the last passenger from my flight welcomed into India.

Occasionally someone would nod in my direction and speak to another official. Finally a potbellied bureaucrat strode into the room, glanced at me, and reached for the telephone. He murmured something about the Indian Home Ministry into the receiver. I held my breath as I heard my name spoken amidst a flurry of Hindi syllables. An unidentified voice on the other end of the line growled, and this man repeated the order: "Yes, sir. Refused entry." The needle screeched wildly across the vinyl.

> *I did not think, on this wintry night, you would come.*
> *You came near, and still nearer and all the doors were closed*
> *Not even once did I ask you inside*
> *On this rainy wintry night.*

For most of the 1980's I had lived in Asia, studying and working with the yoga and meditation organization, Ananda Marga, that Sarkar had founded. After the first several years, captivated by his practical approach to connecting with spirit, and though I never would have believed it possible before coming abroad, I decided to become a monk. I saw this as a commitment to something beyond my own eternally needy self: a life of strict daily practices, of actively loving God. And it had clicked for me—I'd been swept happily along within a magnificent current of grace and clarity.

Sarkar was deeply interested in the connection between spirituality and social justice. In the early 70's, critical of the Indian government for its inability to address the country's crippling poverty, he'd put forward an ambitious agenda geared toward restructuring the economy, with a focus on cooperatives to generate purchasing power for the poor. This radical commitment must have stirred strong resistance from the establishment; his organization, along with others, was banned during the mid-70's, a period known as India's "Emergency" when then-Prime Minister Indira Gandhi implemented martial law. As a result, Sarkar's foreign followers sometimes found themselves blacklisted by Indian immigration.

I, too, had been deported from India in the mid-80's and some shadow of this event, I guessed, was the problem now. Yet it had been fifteen years since I'd left Asia; I'd assumed that lawsuits brought on behalf of other foreigners against the Indian government would have changed the policy, since it was technically illegal to deport people on religious grounds. Or, given India's unwieldy bureaucracies, that such a blacklist would blow off a table or molder in the heat or get lost in some musty storage room in the Home Ministry.

But on this night, India surprised me. Beautiful things always have a mixed nature—this I'd discovered before. Though I was here as a scholar, it made no difference. Less than two hours after arriving in

Bombay, I was escorted back onto the plane to Milan, unceremoniously booted out of the country.

As I boarded, the Alitalia airlines liaison, an Indian man, saluted me mournfully: "Sir, very sorry my government is doing this to you."

"I'm sorry, too."

The mother of an Indian friend in Bombay had arranged a train ticket to Calcutta for me, a ticket that would now go to waste. She was waiting for me to contact her, but of course I could not. My friend later told me that her mother, on learning that I was refused entry, worriedly asked: "What? Is he some kind of terrorist or something? What kind of friends are you having, anyway?"

On the flight back to Chicago I sank into my seat, exhausted and angry. I would have to explain things to the foundation which had awarded me the grant, but I couldn't yet wrap my head around it myself. The deportation was a reminder of a historical tension in India. But it was also more personal. It was in India that I'd embraced something deep; the place had become a spiritual home for me. I'd wanted to return to India, also, because some mysteries needed solving. The organization Sarkar founded had, after his death, begun to fragment. I'd hoped, in coming to India, to get a better sense of where things were headed, to shore up my faith in this vision. Now I'd been turned away, and it wrenched my heart.

The tiny lights in the ceiling of the cabin began blinking off one by one. Trying to relax, I let my mind wander. I thought about my journey, my adventure, begun some two decades ago. It had not simply been a trip through time and space, roughing it across the great cities of Asia—beginning in Bangkok, and on to Tokyo, Seoul, and of course, Calcutta.

It had been, when you came right down to it, a journey toward a new self.

PART ONE — BANGKOK

CHAPTER ONE

Golden stripes of sunlight danced across the wall as I sprawled on the hard wooden floor of the Bangkok yoga center and snuggled inside my sleeping bag. Strange sounds drifted up from the street, the jangly tonal vowels of the Thai language—like spoons dropped on a concrete floor—schoolchildren teasing each other, a man and a woman quarreling, hawkers on bicycle carts bleating their signature cries for fruits and sweets: "*PHOONNN LAAAA MAIIII!*" As I blinked myself more fully awake, an understanding dawned in me that, on this sunny morning, I was awakening in the heart of Asia, far from home. Possibility folded around me like an origami crane.

I'd arrived in Thailand the day before, shouldering my backpack and strolling out of Don Muang Airport in a state of Christmas morning wonder. A strong wave of humidity washed over me as I exited the air-conditioned terminal. Several taxi drivers pounced. "Many, many discount," one promised, smiling broadly. I loaded my pack into the trunk of his aging sedan, and we zoomed toward the city, past first glimpses of tropical Siam: fields of vibrant green paddy and palm trees beneath pregnant clouds billowing against the bluest of skies.

Buddhist temples in the distance shimmered orange, red and green, like Oz's Emerald City. We drove past stands of fruit the likes of which I'd never seen before—blue bananas (*blue bananas!*), torpedo-shaped papayas, the spiky *durian* that my driver claimed "taste like heaven but smell like hell!" Throngs of people clogged the streets and sidewalks, driving *tuk tuks*—those ever-present three-wheel cabs—and taxis, selling bitter melons and bananas, doing what people do, but in a manner utterly new and fascinating to me.

Bangkok's official title is also the world's longest: "Great City of Angels, Supreme Repository for Divine Jewels, Great Land Unconquerable, Grand and Prominent Realm, Royal and Delightful Capital

City full of Nine Noble Gems, Highest Royal Dwelling and Grand Palace, Divine Shelter and Living Place of the Reincarnated Spirits."

The fare of my beaming taxi put me back $40, which I later learned was more than four times the standard rate.

The next day dawned clear and fair, and the Indian monk who'd welcomed me the previous night, all twinkling eyes and unruly beard, peered at me over the scattered remains of our Bangkok breakfast. An elfin young man with long black hair, clad in a saffron gown, he suggested a walk. Slipping his hand into mine, he led me out through the metal gate in front of the house. The heat and oily humid smells conjured some vague memory, perhaps of mowing lawns when I was a kid.

We strolled back and forth in the lane through the perpetual summer of Bangkok as cars and tuk-tuks whizzed by on the nearby thoroughfare.

"Tell about yourself."

I told him I had come to Thailand to look into working at a school for poor kids. I didn't tell him that I had also come because I couldn't see beyond the black hole of my own self and that I had needed to get away from the States in order to clear my head. "Oh, Andy," a friend who fancied herself a palm reader had murmured not long before, taking my hand and searching the patterns of my palm. Weighing my hand in hers, and noting the plethora of tiny scratches from broken main lines, not deep and smooth, but full of false turns, fibrillations, breaks, cul-de-sacs, she looked up.

Pushing her hair out of her face, she sighed: "One rough ride."

I couldn't argue. In my late teens there were days when I'd imploded, couldn't bear to be around other people, couldn't throw a single spark of personality beyond the horizon of my depression. The default ways in which males in my culture were encouraged to become men—sex, drugs, wildness—had left me confused, though I had tried them on for size. I'd been traditionally churched among Presbyterians, but at a certain point this, too, had left me cold, and I found myself turning away from the faith of my fathers. There seemed to be no real rites of passage in my world, no means to understand what it was to become whole. At age 21, I was entering a life, as T. S. Eliot had put it, of being "distracted from distractions by distractions."

The monk smiled at me. Perhaps he could read the general outlines of my dilemma in my face. "This life is not easy," he said in his nasal, high-pitched voice. I stared at him.

"As a monk, I am surrendering everything for a higher purpose, giving up everything, for God. So, I am able to be..." he searched for the word... "concentrating completely on service, and on meditation."

He turned his doe-eyes to me. "Do you think you could do like this?"

I gave a nervous laugh. It was something I hadn't really considered. And besides, I had just gotten here. I wanted to explore and enjoy. I wanted to have some fun.

"Think about this," he said. "You are inviting a friend to your house. Are you keeping the door closed? No, you are opening it."

He laid his hand on my shoulder.

"Open yourself."

We came to a crosswalk, and stood waiting for the light to change. Of course, I did want to believe that I had untapped potential within me. But I also didn't want to have to give anything up. I was in Thailand for just a year, I reminded myself, to undertake a grand adventure, get my act together, and learn something about the world. That was all. Wasn't it?

The light changed. And we strolled on, hand in hand, under the blistering Bangkok sun, while the monk affectionately cracked my knuckles.

I'd been living in Austin—this was 1982—half-heartedly attending the University of Texas. There I had learned to practice meditation, and there I happened to meet a yogic nun, Didi Ananda Mitra, who was passing through town. A brilliant and enthusiastic scholar, she had embraced the yogic path, committed herself to following a guru, and written extensive commentaries on this master's teachings.

Perhaps she perceived my restlessness. "I've spent a lot of time in Southeast Asia," she told me. "In Bangkok we're trying to open a school for poor children. Why not go there and help out?"

Just like that. *Why not go to Bangkok?*

Spinning the blue-green globe I kept on my bookshelf, watching the multi-colored blur of countries slip by, I savored the sounds of Asian cities on my tongue: Bodhgaya, Kwangju, Kuala Lumpur. Shinchu, Cebu, Pattalung. My finger traced the route I might take, over the North Equatorial Current, the Tropic of Cancer, the great bulge of China, on to the slender appendage that was Thailand.

Bangkok held various attractions for me, but it also happened to be the city where a favorite writer of mine, the Trappist monk Thomas Merton, had died in a freak accident while on a pilgrimage to the East.

He had just been to India and Sri Lanka where he'd had a kind of breakthrough at the great Buddhist statues of Polonnaruwa, exclaiming, "I don't know when in my life I have ever had such a sense of beauty and spiritual validity running together in one aesthetic illumination."

Then he addressed a group of fellow monks in Bangkok. "The monk is a marginal person, who withdraws deliberately to the margin of society with a view to deepened fundamental human experience," he told the assemblage. "The task of the solitary person and the hermit is to realize within himself a universal consciousness and to contribute this into the communal consciousness." The next day an electric fan fell onto the wet floor as Merton dried himself after a bath—electrocuting him. Ironically, his body was flown back to the U. S. with the bodies of servicemen killed in Vietnam.

I was intrigued by Merton's linking of spiritual and social concerns, his thoughts on monastic life, especially as I knew I would be living with monks if I came to Bangkok. Though Thailand was primarily a Buddhist country, the meditation practiced at the center where I would be staying wasn't Buddhist. The monks who lived and taught there were yogis, embracing the mysticism at the core of India's spiritual tradition and committing themselves to sharing it with others.

I liked the meditation practice and was inspired by the calm demeanor of other yogis I'd met in Texas. My studies at UT were going nowhere; I could always resume them later, hopefully after I returned to the States with more sense of purpose. So I began saving money, taking a part-time job at a Tex-Mex restaurant called Los Tres Bobos, telling my co-workers that I was going to Thailand for a year.

"Damn, man, I should do something like that!" one of them exclaimed. I savored the slight aura of celebrity my upcoming trip generated. My parents were agreeable to the idea of my traveling, too, even donating some money for the ticket.

Travel, I thought, would offer a chance for new energy to percolate through me. I was young, of course, but I could be bold when I needed to be. Time away might be just the thing to pull me out of my doldrums.

The Ananda Marga yoga center in Bangkok stood halfway down a long narrow street, sandwiched between student digs and middle-class homes. Inside, a photo of wild giraffes gamboling on an African plain clipped from *National Geographic* was taped to one of the walls. This was the Indian monk's effort to spruce things up a bit. Otherwise, the décor was sparse. No television. No sofas or chairs. If I wanted to read, I rolled up a blanket, placed it under my head, and lay with a book on the upstairs wooden floor. At mealtimes, we spread newspaper on the concrete floor downstairs, and gathered cross-legged around this makeshift tablecloth.

I'd come prepared, mostly, for this spartan existence. The little I'd brought with me from the U. S. was more than enough for my needs: two pairs of pants, four shirts, my father's Zeiss-Ikon single-lens reflex, Hawthorne's *Twice Told Tales*, a small cassette player, and a copy of Cat Stevens' *Greatest Hits*.

Openness to simplicity, I discovered, would serve me well here. The monks had a word for this. They called it *aparigraha*, which translated roughly from the Sanskrit as "treading lightly on the earth." Living so that you weren't contributing to the poverty of others, not amassing too much *stuff*. This appealed to me, especially as I began to see how these monks put their ideals into practice.

Besides the Indian, there was a German monk living here, a multifaceted man with eyes that were deep and serene, who'd been a student of Chinese philosophy before becoming a yogi. An intellectual, he enjoyed discussing the subtleties of yoga philosophy. But he had a practical side, too. Haunting junk shops around the city, he trolled for old printing presses or other equipment which he fixed up and shipped off to service projects in other parts of Southeast Asia. Evenings, he played the flute.

"Young friend," he said on meeting me. "You want to be a yogi? I like it very much."

I watched him sit unmoving in the meditation room one morning for two hours straight. Peering in from time to time, I took note of his locked legs, the straightness of his spine. He seemed to have settled so deeply into some impenetrable state of serenity that I, who struggled to sit still for ten minutes at a time, could only watch with amazement.

What else did these men do? They offered free instruction in yoga and meditation, engaged in small business ventures to support the center, and organized mass feeding projects in the slums. They were members of an international movement promoting spirituality and social justice. And as other members of this meditation group arrived from Hong Kong, Sydney or Los Angeles and spent a day or two in Bangkok before heading on to the headquarters in Calcutta, the monks played host to these travelers as well.

On one of those first mornings in Bangkok, heat lightning flared across the sky, presaging a storm, and I decided to scrap my elaborate tourist plans. I sat shyly on the back porch with the two monks—the Indian dressed in his saffron gown, and the German in white undershirt and orange sweatpants. Behind the house a sea of wastewater weeds floated into the countryside. The Indian encouraged me to address them by the informal term, *Dada,* a Bengali word meaning "respected elder brother," much easier to pronounce than their actual multi-syllabic Sanskrit names.

I told them I was interested in helping at the school the yogic nuns, or *didis,* were starting. "That's good," Indian Dada said. But, he added, the school was far from being ready to open.

I didn't know what to make of this, and so sat in silence for a while, listening to the plinking of rain on the corrugated tin roof. The rain showed no sign of letting up, and German Dada suggested we spend our time productively. He wanted to explain something to me about the history of yoga. Whenever an idea particularly excited him, he punctuated his explanation with the phrase, "I like it *very* much."

"The term 'yoga' comes from the Sanskrit root *yunj,* meaning to yoke or unify," he began, peering at me over the rims of his glasses. "Union with what? Or rather, with whom? With God. Yoga appeared as a revolution in Indian thought. It was an alternative to the purely external Vedic rituals and sacrifices that marked India's early religious development. It internalized the ritual of relating to the divine, you see, focusing on ways to know God within oneself. I like this very much."

With a rush and a howl the wind blew needles of rain onto the porch. German Dada was on a roll. "The meditation practice of yoga, known as *raja yoga,* is nested within a larger tradition synthesizing several approaches to realizing God: we have *karma yoga,* finding God through work and service to others, while remaining unattached to the fruits of your actions. Then there is *bhakti yoga,* the path of love and devotion, and *jnana yoga,* finding God through study and knowledge. I like it very much. But if you ask me what I like best, I would have to say the path of love. It's here that the heart finds its deepest fulfillment." And he beamed.

I listened, while scattered pools of rainwater behind the house began to expand and merge. We watched as a flotilla of paper cups, slippers, a nest of sticks and branches floated by. Suddenly, with startling swiftness, two feet of dirty water coursed through the streets. The neighborhood was flooded.

German Dada sprang up and ran downstairs. Sure enough, water had begun to crest into the first floor of the house. He called us down, handed out brooms and long-handled squeegees, and we mopped at the floodwater, trying to push it back out the door. From his manner I gathered this kind of thing happened pretty regularly. After half an hour of splashing, I leaned on my broom, panting, my shirt clinging to my back. I hadn't expected to spend one of my first days in Asia raking muddy rainwater across a concrete floor.

But Indian Dada smiled at me broadly. My companions seemed to see this as all in a day's work. I gave Dada a sheepish grin. Then, stepping out into the front courtyard, I turned my face to the sky, my toes squishing in the mud, and let the Thai rain sink into my skin.

Chapter Two

I had big plans for this sprawling city. One day I hopped a bus downtown, where, from dark tunnels of shops enshrouded by canvas awnings, the sound of haggling reverberated— *"Mai dai, mai dai!"* Mysterious commodities were to be had: barrels of twisted curative roots, jars of preserved toads or snakes, oversized mushrooms hanging in clumps, along with bootleg cassettes of Madonna and AC/DC, and tubes of "Darkie" toothpaste with their unfortunate depiction of a minstrel in blackface displaying sparkling white teeth.

The Chao Phraya river dissected the city, as wide as the Mississippi in some places. Rolling on from mysterious points north— upper Thailand, Cambodia, China—muddy, choppy, yet full of little ferries carrying passengers through tangles of asparagus-green weeds to the other bank. On one side sat prestigious Thammasat (Place of Dharma) University, where not long before students had protested the latest in a seemingly endless series of military coups, and then, to avoid being shot by advancing riot troops, they leapt into the river.

In the floating markets, women in straw hats paddled their long-prowed boats loaded with green vegetables up to the dock. The plump vendors laughed when I trotted out the few words of Thai I'd picked up. I smiled back at them, finding freedom in not being known, in this quirkiness of having few responsibilities.

The woks of noodle joints smoked and spattered on the bank, proprietors frying chilis amidst a great whoosh of steam while barefoot boys ran between the tables. As night came on, lanterns were set out, strangers became dining companions, and the pungent smells of the sea floated up the river.

Heading home at the end of the day, I strolled past a little shop on our lane where I discovered you could buy a fantastic soymilk. Sitting at a table outside the shop I sipped the cold milk, nodding to our Thai neighbors in the zero-lot line houses.

Everything was exciting, everything exotic, and all of it, I felt, had been placed here for me to discover, and for the liberating effects which its discovery would have on me.

A chubby Thai student named Suraviit was a frequent visitor at the yoga center. One morning he asked if I'd like to visit a reformed Buddhist temple he knew about. I was game.

We took a bus to an outlying district and got off in front of a modest building where small immaculate huts ringed the perimeter of a main administrative center. Inside we sat on straw mats on the wooden floor among a crowd of lay Buddhists, and sweated slightly from the heat. An aged abbot tottered in and delivered a long sermon in Thai, through which I fidgeted politely. When he finished, in scurried a horde of tiny but agile Buddhist grandmothers who laid out dish after tasty vegetarian dish on the table. I glanced at Suraviit, who grinned back at me. This, apparently, was the real draw.

As we ate, Suraviit translated for me the gist of the monk's talk, in passable if convoluted English.

"Don't hold, or better say, don't cling, to old, how to say concept of yourself."

I nodded, reminded that hovering at my shoulder were a number of phantoms stoking a long-time melancholy I would be more than glad to be rid of, though I wasn't sure how to go about it.

Two years earlier, I'd stood alone on the roof of a 20-story dormitory in Austin, my fingers grasping the chain link fence as I gazed across the city. In the distance, the monumental sweep of the Longhorn football stadium, the stately LBJ library, and a string of cars whizzing by on Interstate 35. I was thinking about how easy it would be to simply climb the fence, close my eyes, and then drop. My body would fly past the windows and shocked faces of schoolmates, casting a rapidly growing shadow over busy Guadalupe Street. Then it would all be over.

I felt cut off, anguished, unable to find my place in the world. Perhaps this sense of disconnection was a result of growing up a sensitive soul in Texas with its rough, dog-eat-dogie ethos. Or perhaps it was simply something I carried within me from long back, a seed that demanded to be seen through to fruition, whether that end be bitter or sweet.

But something else had loomed in the back of my mind that day on the roof, some unknown quantity counseling patience. Not a voice whispering restraint exactly; perhaps a kind of prescience, an understanding that things had to get better. My coming to Asia could be part of this process.

Suraviit and I continued to enjoy the feast. Soon a young Thai, his hair cropped short, approached our table. He smiled at me and said, "You like see pretty beauty flower?"

Huh? I followed him toward another building, and we climbed the stairs to a small wood-paneled room. In a long rectangular glass box at the center of the space lay a dead girl. Startled, I moved closer.

She was maybe eighteen, and a floral print dress was smoothed across her body, a sprig of some tropical flower pinned on her breast. There was a delicacy in her small arms. Despite an open window, the air seemed to have been sucked clean out of the room. In one corner a fly buzzed listlessly, then was still.

I tried to decipher my guide's casual manner, wondering what had moved him to bring me here. It seemed clear this was a kind of set piece displayed to visitors. It didn't much matter who the girl had been. Hers was a cautionary tale. Pretty Beauty Flower had died young and unexpectedly, and it could happen to any of us, at any time.

The Thai boy cleared his throat. "All die. Better no attach things."

The room was a little creepy, but I took the point. Nothing stays the same; everything is in flux. The body, too, is only temporary.

It hit me then that I was moving through a different world, a place where pains were taken to remind you of the ephemeral nature of things. Pretty Beauty Flower's message got me thinking. What was I going to do with the time allotted to me? Sure, I was young, but what was the span of a human life, really? A flicker in the dark. I wanted to be useful, for my life to have meaning. I wanted to leave a footprint on the world.

The problem was this: it wasn't death I was afraid of.

The routine at the yoga center, or *jagrti*—the Sanskrit term the monks used—included meditation four times a day. I began to take advantage of this chance to sit regularly with others. Getting up at five each morning, I shuffled downstairs to the candle-lit meditation hall. Sleepy and stiff, I chafed at the discipline it required, but slowly the ritual became something I looked forward to. Folding my blanket into a rectangle, I'd cross my right foot over my left thigh, and twist my back to coax a satisfying pop from my spine before lining it up straight. Then, folding my hands in my lap, I'd roll my tongue against the curved palate of my mouth, and close my eyes to the world.

I'd had a few deep experiences with meditation in Austin. But meditating with monks in this dedicated environment was something different. As if I was piggybacking on their energy, I found it much easier to concentrate. Sometimes it felt as if I were slipping my mind into a cool, comfortable bed with freshly laundered sheets. Meditation, I was coming to see, was a way of stripping down, letting go, if only for a few moments, of obsession and worry, of all thought, really, and settling into deep contentment. I wanted more. Though I wasn't sure if it were possible, I wanted to feel this way all the time.

And so, four times a day I sat, observing the long, sinewy webbing of my inhalation and exhalation. My breath dropped like an anchor through my mind's rough sea of distractions. What we practiced— what I was learning to practice—here was not meditation as stress reduction, or yoga as a way to lose weight or build body strength. It was something more radical, more far-reaching, and as far as the original intent of yoga was concerned, more fundamental. It was *sadhana*—the effort to merge one's *atma* or individual soul, with *paramatma*, Cosmic Soul.

I'd come across a newspaper article entitled "Yoga—is it enough?" questioning whether the stretching of yoga was a sufficient workout, or whether it needed to be supplemented with aerobic exercise. One might as well ask, "Communion with God—is it enough?" The traditional goal of yoga—to prepare body and mind to come closer to spirit—seemed often overlooked. In Bangkok, I began to appreciate this contemplative goal.

Of course, during meditation my mind went traipsing down every back alley of memory and musing that rose before it. My thoughts veered into neurotic monologues: *Hey! Look at me! Look at how straight my back is.* Conversations from earlier in the day replayed themselves, as I tried to winnow out some clever response I could employ later. I was used to judging everything, and judging myself as well. *This is cool, this is stupid.*

But when I was able to release my tight grip on this habit of judgment and simply nestle into consciousness, something remarkable happened. Meditation seemed to open up some space within, loosen some rusted bolts, like an application of mental Liquid Wrench. It seemed to be creating the space for me to grow into something new.

As German Dada might have said, "I like it very much."

The school that I'd been invited to help in Bangkok was, as Indian Dada had mentioned, far from ready to open. I did begin preparing materials, following the lead of a British nun who lived a few miles away and whose assignment was to get it off the ground. But there were many obstacles. I'd assumed I would leap right in, but the desire to do good came smack against a lack of funds and training. In a few years, this organization would build what would become a very successful school, reaching out to the poorest children of northern Thailand. But apparently the time was not yet right.

Still, I wasn't married to the project, especially since there was plenty else to do. I began taking on more responsibilities at the jagrti. I also began teaching English to Thai teenagers at a private academy on Silom Road. After a few nerve-wracking initial sessions I settled into the teacher role, standing at the front of the classroom, extracting English phrases from the students. I began to like the work. And my students liked me. One of them, a tiny eighth grader with a beaming, innocent face, invited me to speak to her junior high school class.

So one afternoon I crossed the Chao Phraya by ferry and was met by the girl and her giggling uniformed schoolmates on the far side. They escorted me to their school, where I rambled on to her class about the differences between Thai and American culture, fielding questions on John Travolta and Gloria Estefan for half an hour. Afterwards, the girl took me to a restaurant for soymilk with her friends.

"I am Christ-ian," she said in her careful English. "And you?"

"I, well, my family is Christian. I'm very interested in Eastern religions. I practice yoga."

"Ohhhh, yo-ga."

We sipped our drinks and chatted a bit more.

As we parted she beamed, "I will pray to Yo-ga God for you."

Ever since arriving in Asia, I'd run into "believers." In the Taipei transit lounge, where I'd waited to catch a connecting flight to Bangkok, a cluster of Chinese Christians passed their time singing hymns. The words had sounded strange and jangly, but the tunes radiated out from some cubbyhole of familiarity, leaving me touched in an unexpected way, but also a little exasperated. I'd thought I was leaving many things behind when I came to Asia, not the least Christianity, yet here it was again in force.

The religion ran in my blood. My grandfather, father, brother-in-law—all were or had been preachers. And my brother had spent some time in seminary. So naturally it had seeped its way into me, marked me through years of church potlucks, Vacation Bible School, the intercessions of missionary aunts concerned about my soul. Birthday cards from extended family members contained promises to pray for me. Christian language, imagery, the gospel of love and the sometimes stubborn righteousness, all floated in a heady stew that had been served up to nourish my way of thinking.

Long after I gave up going to church, I had sympathies. One night I dreamed I was hitchhiking and got picked up by a van full of Christians. It took me a while to tease out the dream's essential idea: Christians as fellow travelers in this world of spirit. In fact, I still liked the radicals very much: Dorothy Day and the Catholic Workers, Thomas Merton and the mystics, those who embraced fully the challenge at the heart of the Gospel—love without discrimination.

In December I attended a sing-along of Handel's "Messiah" at a Bangkok church frequented by expatriates. There I rose to belt out the "Hallelujah Chorus" with a pew full of other Westerners. And when I was on errands in downtown Bangkok I often did my noon meditation inside the cool sanctuaries of Christian churches. Amidst the noise and heat of the city, I would find a quiet retreat. Bangkok's Presbyterian church left me nostalgic as I sat for sadhana in half-lotus pose on its pews. Anyone who spied me must have thought I was deep in prayer.

In this way, filaments of my upbringing continued to reach out to me. It was as if the invisible guardians of my old life, my old religion, had noticed I was missing and, alarmed, had fired flares into the night sky of my Asian adventure. Search parties might be sent out, but though I made use of the supplies they had left for me, I didn't wish to be found.

CHAPTER THREE

Family Flashback.

My paternal grandfather emigrated from Britain early in the last century, and then served for most of his life in Massachusetts and upstate New York as a Baptist minister. He and my grandmother raised eight children, most of whom adhered to a similar conservative religious life. But I was interested in the exceptions—an uncle who ran away to join the Merchant Marines, an aunt who earned a PhD in history and married a Palestinian.

My father, second oldest child, grew up to marry a Presbyterian, embracing my mother's more liberal faith and eventually deciding to attend seminary and then do missionary work. In the early 60's my parents traveled to the Mato Grosso, a flat, expansive plain cradling Brazil's Amazon valley. Perhaps seized by a vision of a better world, the urge that rings in most every human heart but is often obscured, they left the lives they had known in the United States behind.

In Brazil my mother worked to create a home in the dusty outback, while Dad led services at several small churches, traveling by jeep, and sometimes by horseback, fielding and strengthening Presbyterians in this Catholic country. I was born there in 1961, Missionary Kid, expatriate child, wrapped in the protective layering of faith as tightly as in any baby blanket.

Flying back from the maternity hospital in Campinas to Mutum where my parents were based, the small plane carrying my mother and me bobbled above an ocean of green forest etched by silver ribbons of river, casting its shadow over hectares of banana plantations and coca fields. The pilot swooped low over Mutum, buzzing the main street until people cleared out of the way. Then the plane jerked down on the bumpy dirt plaza, one wheel at a time, with excited children running along in its wake. At the end of the plaza my father stood and waited. At his side, my brother Bill, ten, stood silently, while my sister Susan, seven, squirmed impatiently. My family rushed to the plane and my mother and I were helped from the cockpit. After such an entrance, I'm told I was a favorite among the locals, the women pinching my pink Gringo cheeks and exclaiming, *"Bonitino Andrezinho!"*

Some new considerations may have been afoot in the American church hierarchy in those days, though, in an effort to redress the complicated history of the missionary calling. There began to be a movement within the church, a pulling back from overt evangelization with American missionaries heading up local churches in favor of cooperation with locals.

As a result, my family's travel in Brazil was not a diaspora, but a temporary sojourn. A year after I was born, they returned to the great humming flux of the American middle class. My father was posted as minister first in El Paso, Texas, then to Gibson, Iowa, a town of just 80 people, where I began elementary school. The town's infrastructure stopped where corn and bean fields began and stretched to the horizon. Orange light danced across the soybean tendrils there, each dusky husk shimmering. Wandering among these fields, I felt there was magic in the world, a great mysterious shining thing that promised freedom and delight.

Dad preached at the only church in town, a white clapboard building with stained glass windows on each side refracting sunlight over the faces of the congregants as they worshiped. I enjoyed a proprietary run of the churchyard, and was granted prizes like the chance to combine leftover communion glasses of grape juice and swig them down in one gulp. Like most children, I accepted the beliefs of my family implicitly. Faith seemed to "work." In those early days I felt I belonged.

My parents' faith focused on the Trinity and on following Christ's example, though the espousal of these beliefs was in keeping with a Midwestern small-town sense of decorum: no tongue-speaking, aisle-rolling, or hands raised above waist level. Not much room, in fact, for expression of feeling at all, and this reticence laid down a template for me. As I got older I wanted to be more expressive but didn't seem to have the tools for it.

The church, our place in the hierarchy of it, was unconsciously held out to me as a sustaining force. Without quite understanding how, the PK, Preacher's Kid, participates in something greater than himself—hooked into a larger community, the spiritual needs of neighbors discussed at home.

At the same time, a scrap of conventional wisdom blowing in the breeze would later find in me solid confirmation: the PK is often the wildest child.

In 1974 we moved to Arlington, Texas. It wasn't until years later that I sensed that my father had pursued a religious life, in part, to live up to his own father's expectations, and that after grandfather died, perhaps my dad wanted to strike off on his own. But it was a bumpy transition, and for a few years after we moved he was unable to secure a decent job.

It was back in Texas that, with the blurred intensity of a cattle stampede, my life turned upside down. Plopping down into this strange new world as I was about to enter seventh grade where my knowing no one was a tough gig. And my father, too, seemed more distant, as if living under that wide sky placed him at another remove. He often retreated into his study, leaving me to wonder what he was thinking in there.

The long-haired boy who planted himself in front of the gym showers at Hutcheson Junior High and began snapping his wet, tightly-rolled towel at the thighs of any kid foolish enough to brave his gauntlet, epitomized the prevailing mood. His behavior seemed part adolescent cruelty, but also part glimpse into the new masculine paradigm, especially in Texas: *Boys, you're on your own.*

So I looked to church for support. First Presbyterian Arlington had a large, well-heeled congregation, a departure from the cornfield simplicity of Dad's earlier churches. I joined the youth choir and made some friends. On Sundays we trooped into the sanctuary and filed to our places beneath the stained glass representations of Saints John and Paul. And when the moment came to perform, we rose and poured our hearts out, voices rising and rolling off the sanctuary rafters in harmony. Music seemed to accomplish what the rest of the service, for me, did not: it offered an inkling of, an access to, some greater power.

After the anthem, however, slouching behind the high choral loft wall, my friends and I soon reverted to scribbling notes to each other on church bulletins and reenacting in whispers the John Belushi sketches we'd seen on TV the night before. I was being pulled into a new relationship with the church, one that tempered earnestness with irony. In the sanctuary's rarefied atmosphere, spontaneous adolescent laughter was forbidden, which is probably what made it so contagious.

I'd recently begun to wonder about some of the tenets of this faith I'd been bequeathed. Why was it due to *my* sins that Christ had to die on the cross? And why was there so much emphasis on *believing*? Why couldn't you just be open to a spirit of awe and beauty in the universe, without having to submit to some experience that divided people into categories? A youthful skepticism began to take hold.

So that by the time I turned 16, Sundays had taken on a dual character: after singing in the service, my choirboy friends and I flung our robes into the closet and raced out to our cars. We were seeking thrills, which began to involve an excessive combination, not uncommon for young Texans, of beer, marijuana, and staying out all night.

Our behavior was an act of defiance, but also of self-definition, even as it was a means of self-obliteration. As far as I knew, no one else in my family had dabbled in these vices. But I had a burgeoning streak of rebellion in me. I was tired of being good.

One night after choir practice I slipped into the church sanctuary and stood alone beside the gleaming wooden pews. Wine-red carpeting stretched toward the minister's pulpit. The pipes of the organ rose in shiny, orderly rows and the room was bathed in the soft glow of moonlight. The creed that rolled through that space every Sunday echoed in my brain. *I believe in the Father, Son and Holy Ghost, the communion of saints, the forgiveness of sins, the resurrection of the body.*

An image of my grandfather materialized before me. Standing at the pulpit of his Cape Cod church, he cast a shadow of expectation across the generations. I thought, too, about my father. Like many of his generation, he provided for his family, but was at a loss relating emotionally. The distance this created was one I couldn't run on my own; it was of marathon length, and my energy was geared only for quick frenetic sprints.

In those days I wanted to yell at my father, but I remained silent. It wasn't a silence out of which insight could bubble up, not the silent fullness of consciousness as I would discover later in meditation, but an empty silence of self-suppression.

I couldn't know that at that age that all my wildness was really a desperate running after some kind of meaning. As I turned and walked out of the sanctuary that evening, I began searching, deep down, for a spirituality that I could live with.

CHAPTER FOUR

The monsoons blew by, and sunlight streamed through the windows of the Bangkok jagrti. Each morning I placed a blanket on the wooden floor and sprawled like a jellyfish in the tropical warmth. Lying on my stomach, arms at my side, palms down, I enjoyed the feel of the heft of my body pressing through the blanket onto the floor.

I'd put this body through a lot in the last few years, and yet, until recently it seemed I'd been basically unaware of its capabilities. Inching my fingers out next to my shoulders, with a slow sipping in of breath I ratcheted my torso toward the ceiling. Vertebra by vertebra, back and abdominal muscles stretched expansively, imitating the movements of a cobra for which this exercise was named.

A visiting monk from New Zealand talked me through the twistings and stretchings of yoga poses or *asanas*, his gentle Kiwi voice offering snippets of insight into the yogic way: "There is in the body a vital energy. Learn to respect and use that energy.

"Seek balance in all things."

I liked to fold my body first into *janushirasana*, the head-to-knee pose. As I reached down to grasp my toes, I sensed my back muscles loosening, my hamstrings limbering. Strangely, my skin seemed softer, too, since I'd begun doing these exercises.

Rising into the tree pose, I drew one leg slowly up, foot crooked into my groin like a willowy branch, my hands reaching for the ceiling as I swayed back and forth, playing around the edges of that sense of balance which Dada described.

I experienced a satisfying sense of straightness, my body a plane, as I placed my hands against my lumbar and propped my legs and back into the air in *shoulderstand*. Moving into the complementary position of *fish*, my legs folded into lotus, I arched my back like a stone bridge and the crown of my head made contact with the blanket. It felt fantastic!

My stomach had been weak for some time. Dada charted out a set of asanas for me to practice that he said would address this problem. The *peacock*—balancing on my hands as my elbows pressed into my abdomen, my body hovering parallel to the floor—was one of these, and it seemed to help.

Fish. Spinal Twist. Plough. Turtle. Bridge. The evocative names hinted at what the movements looked like from the outside. But implicit in asana practice was an internal benefit, a massage of the organs, meant to stimulate and help the endocrine glands do their thing. As German Dada explained, "These glands secrete and deliver hormones directly into the bloodstream, and asanas exert pressure on them in a positive way."

This, he assured me, would have an impact on my thoughts and emotions, helping me to move beyond identification with lower tendencies, like anger and lust, into higher ones, like self-control and compassion. It made sense to me. Each day as the tropical clouds wafted inland from over the China Sea, a new sense of spaciousness was growing in me. The more I practiced, the calmer I became.

In Bangkok it was all about the practices. And not all of them were easy. One evening Indian Dada caught me by the elbow.

"Tomorrow," he announced, "we fast."

Uh-oh. Overindulgence had been the response I'd mustered to the psychic pressure I'd felt in the last few years. If food was tasty, I ate twice as much as I needed, or was good for me. When I drank alcohol, it was to excess. I indulged in self-pleasure more frequently than desire warranted, in effect manufacturing desire.

To give something up, pare it away—now *that* was a novel idea. Fasting turned on its head the tendency to fill emotional gaps with physical gratification. It freed up energy that was usually channeled into the physical arena, and thus gave you more time to meditate, to work, and to think.

The practice was called (a bit ominously, I thought) a "dry fast": no food, no liquids, from bedtime one night until sunrise on the second day. This gave the digestive tract a chance to rest. There was an ethical dimension to it, too; it was easier to empathize with people who didn't have enough to eat when you knew from experience what it felt like. But I wondered, could I really turn away from food for a whole day and a night?

The next morning the sun rose and began to beat on the city. With a sense of expectation I also rose, bathed and did my meditation. Around breakfast-time my belly sent out its usual rumbling signals. *Hey, it's time to eat.* I ignored this and set to work cleaning the upstairs floor of the house.

By noon, appetite gnawed more persuasively at my stomach and an ache had begun to throb across my temples. I decided to lie down for a nap.

I'd skipped meals before, but never without knowing that another one would soon take its place. I'd spent my childhood indulging sweet and salty taste buds. *Quesadillas* smothered in sour cream line-danced across the screen of my imagination, conjuring the good jalapeno taste of Texas. As the afternoon wore on, the desire to experience the pleasure of a satisfied stomach grew.

After a while all I could think about were the stands of fruit beckoning from the shop down the street. Since arriving in Thailand, I'd cultivated a passion for mangos. I would hold one of the golden varieties in my hand, squeeze it until its insides turned to pulpy liquid, and then break a hole in the top and suck out the sweet, sweet juice.

I could almost taste...it...now.

In the grip of reverie the objects of my desire appeared almost exclusively curved: crescent moon bananas, pregnant pineapples. The state of longing itself seemed to curl round and round, swinging first toward satiation, then toward restraint, in an everlasting S-curve of desire. And still the day slipped by sticky and slow, as if time was made of honey, of molasses, of anything that trickled off the spoon.

I went for a walk to steel my resolve, in the opposite direction from the fruit shop. When I returned, so had the headache. I did a quick evening meditation and went to lie down. Indian Dada had advised me to go to bed early this first time, though I noticed that he himself had had a full day, not slowing down much.

Around eight the longings of the day reached a climax. I could stave off the hunger no longer. The two monks were upstairs reading, so I sidled into the kitchen. Opening cupboards and peering into them as if they were vaults of hidden treasure, I discovered a can of mixed nuts, which I pulled from the shelf. Glancing over my shoulder, I pried the plastic lid off, and with a sigh popped a cashew into my mouth and chewed slowly, savoring the texture. It was tasty.

Then I went to bed, feeling somewhat satisfied, if a little guilty. After a half-hour of restlessness, I fell asleep.

Guilt was never imposed or encouraged by those around me, but there it lay inside of me. Often I felt I needed to sit longer, to rise earlier, to somehow prove myself. And now I felt bad for not sticking to the letter of what was not an easy practice, and this on my first try.

I'd read that Tibetan teacher Trungpa Rinpoche called this tendency to get caught up egoistically in practice 'spiritual materialism.' The ego could as easily get enmeshed in spiritual brinksmanship as in any worldly activity.

Indian Dada, too, had reminded me that spiritual practice should be done with love, not dryly, not mechanically, and certainly not out of a sense of guilt. No specter of hell was ever held out on the yoga path. Still, it took time for me to rid myself of this sense of not feeling "spiritual enough."

But I'd made it through the fast, more or less. And the next morning I felt great, my mind light, my body unburdened. Sitting in meditation, I slipped easily into a state of concentration and forgave myself the forbidden nut.

In the future, this process would become easier. Though it would always take determination, the key to dealing with desire, as I discovered, lay not with my body, but with my mind. If I could engage myself in some constructive work and divert my attention, my desires lessened in intensity until one fine day I discovered a detachment from them had grown like, well, cashew trees in an orchard. This was one of the many blessings of Bangkok life.

Following this path's discipline meant drawing on hidden reserves of strength. The physical environment was tough, too, with the hard wooden floors on which we slept, the sometimes chilly bath water, the ferocity of the bloodsucking Thai mosquitoes. But I was young; I could handle it. Although the life asked a lot, I liked its clear-cut approach, its commitment to service. What had started out for me as therapeutic necessity—a distant light to pull me from my darkness—was slowly building into an abiding spiritual urge. This was an important shift.

That morning, we all gathered in the kitchen, laughing and joking. Birds twittered in the grasslands behind our house. Our neighbors backed their cars out of their garages and drove off to work. I felt closer to the monks, having passed through this trial together. Downing glasses of lemon water and salt to flush out our digestive systems, we enjoyed sweet yellow bananas, and nourished ourselves with yogurt and fresh bread.

I reacquainted myself with mangos.

Most evenings I helped prepare dinner in the kitchen at the back of the jagrti, slicing layers of light green cabbage, dicing potatoes, mincing tiny green chilis. The place filled with steam as Indian Dada, an orange *lungi* knotted above his knees, and with his hairy chest bare, cranked open the valve on the gas canister next to the stove. Pouring bowls of chopped vegetables into a smoking wok greased with peanut oil, he then slipped in small bricks of white tofu and fried them until they were browned.

As we watched the vegetables simmer, Dada crooned an Indian devotional melody. What he lacked in tunefulness he made up for in enthusiasm.

"The food," he explained, "is absorbing the energy of the cook." Chanting or singing ensured that the cooks, the surroundings and those who ate the food were all "properly blessed." What you ate and how it was prepared exercised a subtle effect on your emotional health. If the cook was having a bad day, the perceptive diner sensed it at mealtime. Wiping a few beads of sweat from his forehead, Dada grinned and sighed, "Even rice with a little salt can be a feast. If you are preparing it with love."

There were echoes here of what I'd read of Zen master Dogen, whose 13th century treatise on monastic cooking cautioned monks to care for each single grain of rice. "Handle even a single leaf of a green in such a way that it manifests the Buddha," he wrote. "This in turn allows the Buddha to manifest through the leaf."

I lay newspapers on the floor of the main room and set down the steaming pot of Thai rice. Then I laid out plates and forks. The front screen door had come undone, and so, hoping to deny entry to the evening's mosquitoes, I latched it shut. As I returned to the kitchen to wipe clean the chopping block, I realized that this was the idea I longed to understand: We make the world sacred through our intentions.

Chapter Five

The afternoon sky was tinged with ribbons of color, the sun drifting down through layers of cumulus. My Thai visa had expired, and I was headed to Malaysia to get a renewal. This morning at Hua Lamphong I had boarded a southbound train, which chugged out of the great city and charted down the southern peninsula, passing rubber plantations and palm oil factories, carrying me, along with that setting sun, into the heart of green Asia.

The following week a meeting of Ananda Marga monks and nuns (or *acharyas*, "those who teach by example") from around Southeast Asia was slated for northern Malaysia. I decided that after getting my visa I'd hang out for a week on the margins of this Malaysia conclave. I was looking forward to meeting more of these saffron-clad people.

And after Malaysia? I figured I'd either return to Bangkok, or travel on. Perhaps to India, to see the guru, the man everyone was talking about. His spiritual name was Anandamurti, though he also went by the given name of Prabhat Ranjan Sarkar. The possibility of meeting this man intrigued me, though as yet I knew little about him. Bangkok was a way station really, and though I would live there on and off for more than half a year, I never escaped the feeling of my stay being temporary. If I wanted to go deeper into this practice, India was the place to be.

"My man! Have a drink with us!"

Across the aisle two German 20-somethings shared a bottle of Jack Daniels. With a wink and a raised glass, they offered me a shot.

They were trekking the tourist loop, exploring the Khmer temple ruins and the southern Thai islands. In their cotton drawstring pants and tie-dye shirts they seemed happy to be young and on the road. And for some reason, the drunker they got, the more they wanted to connect with me.

For a moment, I was tempted. Memories of wild nights with Texas friends stirred. Some part of me, albeit a diminishing part, wanted to accept their shot glass. Yet, the more I did meditation, the less I wanted to go back to old habits. What I really wanted was a sense of wellbeing and connection. Couldn't this be achieved without sinking into that bottle? I smiled at the Germans, but shook my head.

Near Haad Yai the train slowed, and we entered the slums on the outskirts of the city. On either side of the tracks small boys congregated. Suddenly a whistle pierced the air. At this signal, the boys pulled water balloons from beneath their T-shirts and gleefully tried to lob them through the open windows of the train cars. One or two balloons made it through, bursting against the floor in a rain of red plastic and water.

Spluttering, the man across from me leapt from his seat and rushed to slam the window shut. Sitting just out of range, I looked out the window and, to my delight, could see the little hooligans rolling on the ground, hooting and high-fiving, as the train pulled us out of sight.

The Germans laughed and offered to buy me dinner, but as I glanced at the dining car menu—prawns, shellfish, chicken—I saw nothing I could eat. Sheepishly, I explained that I followed a vegetarian diet. Again, disappointing them.

One of them frowned. "If you cannot enjoy life, eat what you want, do what you want, what is the point?"

I wanted to say something about how discipline had begun to allow me a *greater* enjoyment of life. But I could tell they weren't really interested. Besides, they had a point. Following this way of life, this path of restraint, did sometimes make it hard to fit in.

Outside the jagrti, I seemed to be constantly justifying myself, my not eating meat, not drinking, the twice or four times daily withdrawal into self. A gap existed between the world of spiritual experiences and noble sentiments expressed at the yoga center, and the work-a-day, skeptical world, taking its pleasure in Saturday night beers at the neighborhood bar. Were these worlds irreconcilable?

I had already felt like an outsider for much of my life. Why, then, should I willingly take on a life of such difference? I would be on the receiving end of this question again in the succeeding years: Why do you do this? Friends were puzzled by the impulse. What's this spiritual practice thing, this meditation and yoga, all about? Aren't morning cups of tea in a sunny kitchen, the touch of a lover's hand, serious work, and the sustaining love of friends and family enough?

Those things were beautiful. Yet I knew there was something more. At this point I could only reference some feeling that had not yet fully blossomed. But I felt that after even the smallest taste of bliss in meditation, the mind opened up in magnitude. It was the moment of experiential truth, a sweet place to be. Hadn't this experience driven the seeker's quest across so many eras? But to most people, who didn't understand the context, it could seem a little weird. And this tension put me on the margins.

On the other hand, as any biologist will tell you, it's in an ecosystem's margins where the richest life occurs.

I shrugged and settled for some buttered bread and cucumber slices. The Germans went back to their bottle.

The train trundled on southward, past the great diminishing forests of Thailand, sparkling white beaches, ghostly hills and villages, headed for the arc of the Malay peninsula. To the east a temple nestled in the hills, its red and green roof tiles shimmering in the heat. Among the trees sat a huge granite Buddha in peaceful quiescence, his hands sculpted into a gesture that seemed to beckon viewers to him.

Around dusk our train lurched across the border, the green hills lining the tracks funneling us into a new country. At Butterworth I transferred to a bus, which shot down the backbone of northern Malaysia. Outside Ipoh bulky rock formations piled up like ragged mounds of dough. Disembarking at the village of Batu Gajah, I shouldered my bag and humped it to the yoga center, for which I had directions. I walked past wooden *kampong* houses raised on stilts above swept courtyards, the smell of salted fish emanating from outdoor kitchens. A hulking water buffalo lolling in a pond looked up as I passed.

Two Indian acharyas with shoulder-length jet-black hair and thick beards stood on the porch of the local jagrti, their orange uniforms ablaze against the white of the house. I was the first visitor to arrive, and these dadas went out of their way to make me feel welcome with a delicious meal of tamarind chutney, *alu gobi* and rice.

One of them kept up a running banter as we ate.

"Are you full?" he asked me. "Or are you fool?" He chuckled, amused with himself. "Ha! It is a play of words."

The other man said little, but his eyes were deep liquid into which I felt I could disappear. Though we had just met, I felt strong affection radiating from him, the sentimental lure of Indian hospitality.

After the meal this quiet man enveloped me in a bear hug. "Andy is good!" he exclaimed. Really? Was I good? I felt the snags of my old life, pulled by old habits that had led me to be oblivious to all but my own selfish concerns. But to this man, I sensed, everyone was potentially good. I melted into his embrace.

The place sounded a quieter note than the busy thrum of Bangkok. A couple of banana trees presided over the front yard, and the neighbors' wash hanging across the fence whipped in the wind. Inside the house, a small kitchen fronted a large open room. Through the iron lattice on the windows wafted the sharp aroma of jackfruit. The meeting would not begin for a few days, so I helped with preparations, raking brush in the yard as the neighbors, Tamil-speaking folk, sat on a bench and looked on from their compound, pointing out branches I had missed.

There were more members of our yoga organization in Malaysia than in Thailand, perhaps because almost everyone in Thailand was Buddhist. Here, due to the multi-ethnic makeup of the country, people from a variety of backgrounds participated. A little yoga community existed, with its own rituals, friendships, and squabbles. Back in the U. S. some of the yogis I'd met seemed to emerge from the counter-culture; they were often students and hippies. Here, more professional people embraced the practice. These local people were happy to have a young American visiting, and shared me around for meals at each other's houses.

Soon, though, a wave of saffron came crashing onto the shores of this little village. I watched as nuns welcomed each other with folded hands; monks clapped each other on the back. "What's your posting these days? Where are you working? When was the last time you were in India?" One monk rumbled up on a motorcycle, his orange gown flapping behind him in the breeze. Inside, someone set up a table and laid out the latest books on yoga they'd published; someone else laid out photos of the children's schools they were overseeing.

I'd helped clean the center and set in a supply of food, and now I watched as a shift in energy took place. I wouldn't be involved in the meetings, during which the acharyas would discuss their work and chart out plans, but the peripherals—the collective meditation, the food, the deep hanging out—I was looking forward to.

While everyone got settled in, German Dada, my friend from Bangkok, shuffled into the main room, picked up a guitar, and began to strum. It was an unusual tune—jazzy, modulating. The sound drifted through the knots of people talking and laughing and got their attention. Dada danced while he played, one big toe tapping the floor behind him, then the other. Other people slowly joined in; it was, after all, almost time for evening sadhana, and after ten minutes, the room was full of dancers.

I'd sung and danced *kiirtan*, this mixture of devotional chanting and ecstatic dance, every day in Bangkok. It was one of the things that lifted me out of myself most, and helped concentrate my mind before meditation. But doing it with such a large group of people was intense, as if we were generating some giant electromagnetic field of rhythm. We sang the mantra—*baba nam kevalam*, a phrase registering the devotional roots of our practice, evoking love for the divine—over and over, in blissful repetition.

The sweetness of the song began to visibly affect people. One didi in front of me bent her knees fluidly like a whirling dervish, gliding back and forth across the floor, arms raised toward the sky. Her face reminded me of the famous frieze of Teresa of Avila, frozen in a moment of ecstasy.

The tambourine player, however, was slightly off. So much so that a Nigerian monk, acutely tuned to the subtleties of rhythm, slyly tugged the tambourine away from the offender, then awarded it to someone he knew could keep the beat. As soon as this person began grooving, the spirit of the tune changed. Nigerian Dada stopped in his tracks, spun, and jabbed his index finger at the player. "Now you've got it!"

The singing grew more intense. Somebody shouted. People leapt into the air. It was like being in the choir when I was a kid, but richer: a choreography for the longings of the heart. There was no need for belief; simply let go and experience joy.

Our voices echoed across the hall, through the windows, above the jackfruit trees in the back yard, and out into the world. Nigerian Dada, a huge smile on his face, clapped his hands in a polyrhythmic blur. The neighbors, sitting on their porch, were tapping their toes.

CHAPTER SIX

In the evening there was homemade pizza, or "pijja," one monk pronounced as he explained to several other puzzled Indians, "It is an American food." We ate together and watched the sunlight filter down through the hills.

From across the room I recognized someone: Didi Mitra, the nun who had inspired me, back in Texas to come to Bangkok! She smiled and walked over to greet me, and I told her a little about the adventures I'd had since first arriving in Thailand.

"I knew it would be the right move for you," she said. "Surrounding yourself with spiritual people deepens your own practice."

Standing next to this woman I did feel a better nature in myself rising. She had dedicated herself to an ideal, and the commitment sparkled in her eyes. These monks and nuns were like sisters and brothers to each other, a change from how I had thought of women back in the States. There, my relationships with the opposite sex were often underlain or defined by desire. That didn't seem to arise in this context. These women projected a no-nonsense clarity about the fact that they were first and foremost spiritual teachers.

They were also assertive. That evening I happened to enter the room as this didi and her boss, a South Indian monk with a pronounced forehead, stood on the landing and argued.

"I *must* attend the global conference in Ghana!" she declared.

"Your first responsibility is to *this* sector," he responded, "AND, you have to get my permission before you can travel to Africa. You are undisciplined!"

"We'll see about that."

Both arguing vociferously; both so sure of themselves. A friend pulled me aside. "Get a bunch of *avadhutas* together in one room," he said, referring to the senior monks and nuns, "and watch out!" He laughed, raising his eyebrows.

It was something I hadn't thought much about. Here was a well-structured yogic organization with a chain of command and code of discipline. Yet dadas and didis often had dynamic personalities, a strong sense of personal initiative, and sometimes struggled to fit themselves into the constraints of the organizational framework. Later I would come to understand that some Westerners, especially the didis, chafed at the sometimes patriarchal management style of the Indian males who were often in charge. The order's founder had tried to shake up this aspect of Indian tradition. Still, social equality was a difficult concept for some Indian men to grasp. Having grown up with a conservative cultural mindset, they found themselves working within a revolutionary organization, tangling with Western ways of thinking and doing. It made for interesting tensions.

For the most part, though, I admired the way the acharyas supported one another. It created cohesion and seemed to make it easier to get work done. This came across in the stories people told. I think I heard the following that weekend. A blaze, the story went, had swept through the slums not far from the Manila yoga center, leaving many people homeless. Two dadas stood in the driveway watching the diminishing glow on the horizon, listening to the news coming in from the streets.

"We have to do some service. We must feed these people," Dada AR said. To which the second monk (who was now telling the story) replied, "We only have eight dollars. How can we possibly do anything?"

"Don't argue," the first one said. "Go with the flow."

So they spent most of their money on vegetables at a nearby market. On the way home, they stopped to buy two cans of milk and some fresh ginger. The second dada mused, "We're not going to feed many people with that."

"What did I say? Just get in the flow."

Heating up a pot of ginger-infused milk, they carried it to the site of the fire and started doling it out along with the cooked vegetables. After a while a man came up and said, "I am inspired by what you're doing. Here's 100 dollars worth of bread. Can you hand it out?" With a growing sense of serendipity, they gathered the sacks of bread and returned to those camped along the side of the road.

The pair worked through the night, and in the morning they returned to the yoga center. There they telephoned everyone they knew and invited them to help. Some boys who had been sent to collect donations of vegetables returned with twelve full sacks. A car arrived with a 50-kilo sack of rice. Another came with a case of beans. A big pot of rice soup was set to boil. And so it went.

"We served rice soup continuously from early morning until late at night for three days," the dada told us. "Finally, on the morning of the fourth day the government started to distribute food to the victims." The front page of the largest newspaper in the Philippines reported that the two monks and a group of volunteers had distributed milk, bread and soup to 2000 fire victims the first night, then fed 20,000 people over the next three days.

Dada smiled as he zeroed in on his conclusion: "All that with only eight dollars. And of course, a little bit of guru's grace."

There it was, a story combining the willingness to throw one's self into service with a mysterious force helping things along. The lesson seemed to be, when you let go of doubt, of the ego's second-guessing pressure, and simply immerse yourself *in the flow* of doing good, amazing things could happen. A sense of congruence in the universe was hinted at in this story. A part of me still questioned this. *Was it possible for the self to get out of the way, ever?* But I also understood that you could analyze things too much.

In this case, the outcome was also attributed to a subtle force, that of the guru. If the stories about him could be believed, he was someone linked to a deeper reality, someone who could and did use his spiritual power to affect the world. At this point I really didn't know who or what this person was. I was only dipping my big toe into this mysterious flow, but I was not averse to stepping into it more fully, and letting myself be pulled along by its currents.

The sun was bright, the sky blue, and I hopped a bus to Ipoh city center with a new friend, where later we strolled in the marketplace. Valmiki was Filipino, taking time off from his sales job to work for this yoga organization. Like many meditators, he'd taken a spiritual name, something to symbolize a fresh start, this one referring to an Indian devotional poet.

Because it was Ramadan, few Malays were out and about, and those who were steered clear of the tempting odors wafting from bakery carts and sweet shops. Malaysia was populated by Chinese, Tamils, and Malays, and the latter were nearly all Muslim. Valmiki looked Malay, owing to a genetic link among a broad swath of Southeast Asian people, so that when he and I sat at a table and ordered sweet rolls, he drew sullen stares, behind which lay unspoken accusations— "Don't you know this is Ramadan? And don't you know that all Muslims fast on Ramadan?"

I liked hanging out with someone my own age. Short, a little pudgy, his head framed by curly black hair, Valmiki nurtured a love for good food.

"Man, I tell you, they make these fried bananas in the Philippines, rolled in sugar and coconut, deep-fried? You've never tasted anything like it!"

Picking up a newspaper, he flipped to the movie listings. *Indiana Jones and the Temple of Doom* was starting in a few minutes at a downtown cinema. We stared at each other for a moment, grinned, and then bolted for the door.

In the darkened theater Valmiki and I cheered at Indy's narrow escape from a giant rolling boulder; we perked up at his flight over Nepal and freefall plunge into India; and we groaned at the scene of the swaying, half-crazed worshippers. It was a Hollywood take on Indian culture, but we enjoyed the film.

"India's nothing like this," Valmiki said as we left the theater, and then with comic timing added, "It's even crazier."

I laughed.

"But it's a beautiful place," he went on. "And our teacher, Anandamurti, is there. You should go."

"Yeah. Listen, Valmiki, let me ask you something. Everyone's always talking about the guru. The dadas and didis, they're so very enthusiastic. But I don't know, it seems kind of weird to me."

It was his turn to laugh. "I was skeptical, too, at first. But he's the real thing. An enlightened person. He's opened my heart. You'll just have to go and see for yourself."

We returned to Batu Gajah in time for meditation. From the bus stop the lights of the house glowed in the dusk. An Indian raga drifted on the night air. The monks and nuns would all soon be scattering, and for some, it was back to the struggle of difficult postings. But they would also be carrying renewed energy.

We slipped in through the kitchen door. Quiet Dada was rolling out flour for *chapatis*. He looked up and smiled. "Where have you been?"

"At the movies, Dada."

"*Acha*? Playing hooky? Welcome home."

My meditation was great here. In the evenings I wrapped myself in a cotton shawl and sat on the porch beneath the comet-seared sky. There was something I was pondering. I didn't really understand what it meant to "realize God." Acharyas talked about it a lot, but it was abstract to me. The theory was that we were all an expression of Supreme Consciousness, of God, on a path toward oneness, and that through meditation we are able to realize this fact, close the gap, cement the deal.

I meditated, and sometimes felt wonderful, but where did God fit into all of this? How did I open myself to Him, or Her, or It?

Perhaps it was by trying, as a small tract urged, to move into that "excruciating sense of absence and separation which builds up within the contemplative, the searing, burning desires that touch the heart of God."

I liked the poetic sensibility of this. So on this night I first sang kiirtan, focusing my attention, and then sat, trying to feel that longing. And perhaps the timing was right. Slowly, my consciousness became light, unmoored, as if it were taking off on one of the towering cloud formations blowing in from the Bay of Bengal. My mind held great clarity. My heart, too, felt full. I couldn't say what it meant, but when after some time I opened my eyes, I felt an immense love for the landscape spread out before me. It was not only a letting go of mental preoccupation, but something deeper. Perhaps this was a settling into *ananda*, bliss. I walked into the village, mingling with the hawkers squatting in front of their carts, the people strolling the sidewalks in the coolness of the evening, the street dogs. I loved them all.

Was this the presence of God? i didn't know, but for now it was good enough for me.

The next day, however, I cursed in the sweltering heat, resenting the impositions of the vendors as they pressed me in the street. How long does the state of bliss last? How long until neurotic personality kicks in again and divine love dries up in the furnace of daily pressures? Clearly the kind of mental peace I desired was something that needed to be worked at and cultivated with care.

Here was something to which you could devote your life.

Chapter Seven

In Austin once, my attention was drawn to a directory that listed various New Age communities. One of the entries described a group of "bright, upscale, urban, competent" yuppies who were "mediating awesome psycho-spiritual energies, including archetypes, kundalini and mind fusion, while polyfidelitous in a community in Beverly Hills." An adjoining ad declared, "Meditate deeper than a Zen monk, at the touch of a button!"

Such approaches struck me as silly and self-absorbed. People seemed to want their spirituality in serendipitous doses—like discovering a sage pumping gas on a desert highway who dispenses wisdom with his wiper fluid. The structure of discipleship was a high price to pay for the average North American, frontier individualism running hotly in his or her blood. I was probably just as reticent. My recent life in Texas had been rooted in rebellion, but without much to fill the void besides sensuality and a generalized discontent.

But this life I stood on the edges of now offered engagement. Living with the disciplined dadas, I could appreciate the advice of religious scholar Huston Smith, who wrote: "When digging for water, it's better to dig one 60-foot well than ten six-foot wells."

One night near the end of the week in Malaysia, the evening meal finished and the dishes washed and put away, I was lounging with a few of the monks. Later that evening, at midnight, they would be heading off to a graveyard to meditate. I tried to take this in.

Cemeteries were quiet and solitary places and were, of course, associated with death. Meditating in such a place, one of the monks explained, helped you to face your fears.

We talked some more and I asked him whether he missed his earlier life. He only smiled.

"But, Dada," I insisted, "you leave so much behind, and maybe you won't even see your family again. That's got to be difficult."

face fear in graveyard

"You see, we sacrifice some things. But we do that in order to serve a larger family. I love and serve everyone. But I'm not attached to anyone." His eyes shone. "That," he said, "is the way of *Tantra*."

I'd heard this word a few times over the past months, though I hadn't fully understood it. It had something to do with yoga, yet the practice and philosophy of yoga had many layers, and I knew I still had a lot to learn. For one thing, what was this about nonattachment? Did that mean not caring, not getting involved with others? I was a little confused.

I had come across books on Tantric sex in bookstores back in Texas. In those days any popular reference to Tantra in the West focused on this perspective; sex sells, after all. But what these acharyas were talking about had little to do with that. The Tantra which they described was about "sacralization" or "making sacred," seeing the world not as a vale of suffering or an illusion to be transcended—as some philosophies had done, but as the evolutionary expression of the divine.

In one Sanskrit derivation, the word 'Tantra' meant warp or weave, representing the web of existence. It could also be translated as "liberation through expansion." The concept was said to have been introduced by the great spiritual teacher Shiva some 7000 years ago as a practice for especially dark times. Historically, Tantra had often been seen as unorthodox and sometimes as transgressive precisely because it was designed to help you face your fears, particularly the fear of death. Such an outlook led tantriks to pursue practices such as meditating at midnight on the burning cremation grounds.

Another reason for Tantra's controversial reputation may have had to do with the use of metaphorical language describing some of the practices, language which worked on several levels. The so-called "Five M's of Tantra" referred, on the surface, to physical practices, but a deeper meaning could be gleaned by those who understood the text. Thus, *Maethuna* was often parsed as sexual union, but it more subtly referred to the union of the soul with God. Similarly, another 'M' seemed to hint at alcoholic intoxication, though it could also be understood as the intoxicating ecstasy experienced in deep meditation.

"Tantra stands for the cultivation of a fearless, compassionate embrace of every situation you encounter, no matter how difficult," German Dada chimed in, also waiting for the midnight hour of revelation. He took inspiration, he said, from the idea that obstacles forced you to reconsider how you use your energies, to think creatively, to struggle.

Tantra was about throwing yourself into your work and your practice with passion. And that appealed to me. There was an edge to it—fighting against one's own baser tendencies, trying to replace them with sustaining ideals, cultivating a firm determination. Just as the true practitioner of martial arts engendered strength and compassion, the tantric was willing to fight, but knew love was the strongest force.

But there was a catch, German Dada said, because the more involved in the drama of life you became, the more the stumbling blocks of ego—anger, jealousy, pride—got the opportunity to stride onstage. Personalities might butt heads like Bighorn rams, feelings get hurt, self-images splinter. I had come to see how these human tendencies didn't go away when you meditated; sometimes they intensified, as the expression of karma accelerated.

Hand in hand with creative risk-taking, then, had to go surrender, an acceptance of one's limitations rooted in humility. And a steadfast holding to the goal, even as the world, and maybe your own mind, was seized by tumult. Seeing beneath the surface of things to the underlying spiritual reality—perhaps this was really what nonattachment meant.

I gazed around the room at the clusters of orange-clad monks and nuns, who were telling stories or singing. They were in it for the long haul. Sure, none of them were perfect. The other day German Dada had lost his temper when he dropped a tray of printing press type, scattering fonts across the floor. And I remembered Indian Dada arguing heatedly over a minute point of philosophy. For the most part, though, they seemed balanced people. If anything, these human flaws reinforced the idea that anyone could pursue this path. You needn't be a saint.

But you did have to try to follow the rules. Someone put into my hands a copy of the rules of conduct that Anandamurti had asked his disciples to follow. Some of them were very interesting:

> *Bear in mind that you have a duty towards—indeed, you owe a debt to—every creature of this universe, but towards you, no one has any duty; from others, nothing is due.*
>
> *One will not be able to know anything unless one develops the psychology of "I know not." It is the fundamental spirit of a true aspirant.*
>
> *Do not have breakfast until you have finished your meditation in the morning. Likewise, do not take your evening meal until you have completed your evening meditation.*
>
> *Artists are great benefactors of society, hence take active steps for their protection. For example, before enacting a drama or its translation, enough money for a day's maintenance must be given to the author.*
>
> *Do not, on any account, accept or offer a bribe.*
>
> *Businessmen, set aside a percentage of your earnings for the poor.*

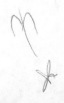

And a list of qualities to cultivate:

Forgiveness. Magnanimity of mind. All-round self-restraint. Moral courage. Keeping aloof from criticizing others, condemning, mudslinging, and all sorts of groupism.

I'd heard that Anandamurti showered his disciples with love and affection, but I also gathered that he was very strict. He knew how easy it was to let things slide. To progress in meditation (and to build a movement), you had to stay focused and follow a certain discipline. This seriousness appealed to me. It was a life circumscribed, yes, but also one shaped and guided into a pleasing form like a bansai tree.

Around Christmas, a year or so earlier, I'd joined other meditators in Austin on a service project. Five of us spent a weekend putting together gift baskets; then we drove around East Austin and distributed them to low-income families. As we made our way through the neighborhoods, the eight-year-old son of one of the women in the car asked, "Can our guru look at something and make it burst into flames with his eyes?"

His mother laughed. "Maybe, but why would he want to? You know, honey, that's not really what a guru is about. The guru helps you to grow, to become a better person."

"Oh," the boy said, somewhat disappointedly.

This woman was effusive in talking about her love for her guru, but it had all been over my head. I liked the people I'd met, and I was beginning to appreciate the practices, but I was pretty sure I had no need of some woolly master.

Yet time in Bangkok had sharpened my curiosity. Visitors passing through lent me books written by this teacher, and I found myself carrying them to a small British library I knew on a quiet downtown *soi* and jumping into them. It was a time of appetite and assimilation for me, of sizing up new ideas. For several years I'd been interested in writers who drew connections between quantum physics and spirituality. I'd learned that Heisenburg spent time with the Indian mystic and poet Rabindranath Tagore, who introduced to him the ideas of inter-connectedness and impermanence as essential aspects of physical reality.

Such ideas were emphasized as well by Anandamurti, who also went by his given name, Prabhat Ranjan Sarkar. Affectionately, people called him Baba, which meant "beloved" or "father." He was writing about some pretty deep things—origins of the universe, the relationship of consciousness and matter, the evolution of mind. Anandamurti had, I gathered, reframed earlier Indian spiritual thought, correcting some perceived shortcomings, adding to it, and contextualizing it for contemporary times.

It was very much a non-dualistic philosophy in which divine substance permeates all things.

God sets the universe in motion by expressing Himself, One manifesting into many. Creation is a curvy affair—waves, rivers, of consciousness flowing through a process of evolution, transforming from Cosmic Mind into matter, the stuff of stardust. Out of matter mind forms. Human beings evolve, and do their thing in the world. It's their *dharma* or essential nature to move toward spirit, and the undulations of their individual minds eventually gravitate toward becoming one with the "straight lines" of Cosmic Mind, the curve of the world's distractions giving way before the pull of the infinite. We move toward God, or sometimes away, but ultimately merge back into that from which we came.

In this framework there is no heaven, no hell, only the clarifying movement of consciousness, yoked to the purifying power of love.

So why did this universe exist? Anandamurti suggested a reason, one which went beyond complicated philosophy and spoke to the heart. Before creation, God was lonely; His nature was to love, but there was no one *to* love. He brought things into being in order to have relationships, especially with human beings, who had the capacity for devotion. He wanted us to come out and play.

But he also wanted us to treat each other right. As Anandamurti, or Sarkar (the name he used when he weighed in on social topics) explained, when you saw that everything was connected, this realization demanded a commitment to human rights and a dismantling of oppressive social structures. Moving beyond the nationalist sentiments of many Indian writers, Sarkar had put forward a more universal vision, calling for the overthrowing of barriers imposed by religion, caste, nationality, and economic inequality.

The slums I'd seen on the outskirts of Bangkok—people living in squalor, falling ill, with little hope—were shocking enough to convince me that something was fundamentally wrong with the way human beings organized themselves. The gap between rich and poor in the world was growing. How many artists, writers or musicians never got the chance to develop their talents due to poverty? How many children never attended school because their families were mired in poverty?

I was thrilled to hear Sarkar declare, "There can be no justification for a system in which a handful grow rich while others starve for lack of a handful of grain."

Handwritten margin notes: "God Cosmic Mind", "God was lonely"

What was going on here? It seemed that Sarkar was leveraging tantric spirituality in order to create movements for radical social change. Don't just live for yourself, he counseled. Think about what you value. Use your energy. Work with others. And bit by bit, help transform the world.

The more I read, the more I appreciated his ideas. At last I'd found a satisfying spiritual and social philosophy, a coherent framework to base my life upon. Taken as a whole, I read it as contributing to a new story, a new narrative about our place in the world. Taking the long view, that humans—like ocelots, like rhubarb, like granite—were originally motes of stardust from ancient blasted novas, infused with varying degrees of consciousness, this story emphasized the importance of interdependence and ecological integrity, of balance in all aspects of life. This was not to say that humans were the same as all other creatures; that would be reductionist. But every being in this world had consciousness, and so all deserved respect and care.

In the 1980's, the extent of ecological devastation the earth faced was not yet clear, but Sarkar knew early on that time was short for the human race to get its act together, to rediscover that balance which might restore both ecological and economic integrity to the planet.

Spelled out in detail in the over two hundred books collecting his discourses and essays, Sarkar's enlightened philosophy lit a fire in my mind.

You could say my real education was beginning.

CHAPTER EIGHT

College Flashback.

My previous education hadn't done much to liberate me. But one class had stood out during my college days. Professor Mackenzie Brown taught a seminar on Asian religions at Trinity University, a private Presbyterian-affiliated liberal arts college poised high on a hill above bustling San Antonio. Trinity was where I began my college career in 1979 and studied for two years, before transferring to the University of Texas.

An eccentric young reed in rumpled corduroy jacket and jeans, medium-length brown hair and wire-rimmed spectacles, Brown looked like he would be more at home tramping the Silk Road than in an academic's office. At the beginning of the first class, he sat at his desk for five minutes without saying a word. When a student raised his hand to ask what was going on, Brown ran to the student, slapped his face, yelled something in Japanese, took off a shoe and put it on his head, and walked out of the room.

Brown fascinated me. As the semester progressed he sat cross-legged on his desk projecting slides of the emaciated Buddha, the *shiva lingam*, the erotic embracings of Indian sculpture, or the Zen sketches of the seeker searching for the ox while riding the ox.

His class was one of several influences in the years before I came to Asia, one that began to open me to a deeper desire for spiritual experience. In fact, a vacuum seemed to be forming in those days, a force field sucking me into some new plane of awareness through the media of my longings.

"Right," Brown would say. "Let's discuss karma, the law of cause and effect. What goes around comes around. As you sow, so shall you reap. This implies an acceptance of the idea of reincarnation—that we all have been here before, that we will be here again, and that there is a reason for all the crap we have to face. That, in fact, we have a hand in creating that crap."

I loved his down-to-earth style, his willingness to grant each of the ideas we studied more than a simple academic nod. I was fascinated by such concepts—ideas people the world over grappled with, embraced or rejected.

Karma, I thought, might go a long way toward explaining why some people were seemingly so free and others tangled up in psychic knots. Certainly upbringing played a role in shaping our psyches, as did family and education, but I sensed that there had to be more to it. Maybe the roles people found themselves playing were karmic extensions? Were our accumulated desires the engine behind all of our restless movement, the longing for love, power or connection compounding itself into a debt that must be repaid?

From an early age I'd felt incomplete. I thirsted for something deeper, almost as if a spark in me were trying but failing to complete an electrical circuit. Maybe it was karma that had brought me to this pass— if not the inborn karma of past lives, then certainly the imposed karma that shaped me in this life. Though I hadn't thought much about the mechanics involved, it made a certain intuitive sense. Every time a person acted, according to this theory, a reaction in potential form was created. This reaction lay within the mind until the proper circumstances arose for its expression. Sometimes that took lifetimes. The mind was like a rubber ball full of indentations, always trying to pop out the dents and regain its former shape.

Later, I would read what one philosopher had written about the *dasein*, "the given," and the journey from the limitations we are born into without choice to the creative freedom of love founded in personal choice and commitment. This was the challenge: to face your karmic momenta or *samskaras*, deal with them gracefully, and begin to live in a way that didn't leave such heavy marks on the psyche.

Two years before I would leave for Asia, I transferred from Trinity to the University of Texas, eager to live in music-hip Austin. My high school church buddy, David, and I would be roommates. We moved into a housing co-op on Nueces Street, a bright yellow Victorian with garrets and spires, called Helios House. Its architectural eccentricities were a good fit for the aging hippies, punk rockers, and open-minded grad students who called the place home for a year or two.

Late into the night David and I would sit in a housemate's room and listen to the timbre of a bamboo flute floating up and around the spires of the house. In those days we all were seeking some slip in consciousness, some shift that would allow us to see the world with new eyes. We smoked, drank, and danced. We filled our heads with Kerouac. Driving through the hill country night in David's muscle car, we listened to the Velvet Underground and the Talking Heads, striving in the best Beat tradition to go beyond our limitations. "Nothing in excess," Aristotle prescribed, but life as a young Texan seemed to require a state of constant excess.

We had fun, and yet sometimes I wandered the streets of Austin, past the egg roll vendors and homeless grifters, not quite having the words to express the thoughts rattling around in my head. *Is there meaning in the universe? Is there anything outside of us?*

The anxiety and depression I'd danced around the edges of in high school soon descended over me like a black veil. Sometimes I felt like a refugee, stomping across the gray sidewalks of campus, doggedly bent on making it to my classes, though not sure what good it was doing me. A scowl shrouded my face, tiredness radiating from my eyes. I often saw the same in the faces of those I passed.

If you have a "why" of living, Nietzsche wrote, you can put up with any manner of "how." This was the problem that dogged me. *Where was my why?*

Amidst the darkness there were moments of clarity. One morning I rode my ten-speed down to the sweeping valley of the Colorado River that flowed past the gleaming state capitol building and out into the brushy hill country. Morning sun enveloped the houses on the eastern bank, and a ghostly film of mist hovered over the water. On the other bank a lone poplar, the crescent leaves on its short branches metamorphosing in color, gained life in the light.

Two bands of ducks rooted through the grass for seeds. Suddenly, as if startled by a noise, they lifted en masse and glided across the water, skimming the surface. Watching, my mind became quiet. Time seemed to slow. I felt they and I were on two ends of the same invisible string. Beating their wings, they formed a single organism with a single intensity, arcing across the river, leaving a rippling trail in the water behind them. Standing silently on the bank, I entered into a sublime stillness that hinted of deeper things. I didn't want to speak, or see another person, only to bask in the changed mood, to let the immensity of the world fill me.

"And I have felt a presence that disturbs me with the joy of elevated thoughts," Wordsworth wrote, as if for me on that bank, "a sense sublime of something far more deeply interfused. Whose dwelling

is the light of setting suns, and the round ocean and the living air, and the
blue sky, and in the mind of man; a motion and a spirit, that impels all
thinking things, all objects of all thought, and rolls through all things."
From time to time, I felt this, too.

Since my introduction to Eastern thought in Mackenzie Brown's
class, I had begun to read, widely, in Buddhism, Hinduism, and Taoism.
I drew a lot of inspiration from this reading, but the ideas were still
mostly abstract to me. I longed for something more practical. So when a
yoga class was offered on the UT campus, I jumped in headfirst. The
class was led by a middle-aged nurse with a Sanskrit name and a gentle
voice, who guided us through the poses and movements with grace.

After several weeks of attending this class I found myself
experiencing my body in a completely new way, my back becoming
suppler than the usual knot of stressed-out muscle tissue. I even felt
a difference internally, as if a flow of blood clear as a mountain rill
coursed through my arteries. It was remarkable. Everyone in the
class seemed to be riding a wave of endorphins. When one woman
blurted out: "This is better than sex!" I could only agree.

I was intrigued by the idea of learning meditation. So when our
instructor announced that a traveling monk was passing through town, I
headed down to the public library to check him out.

In the basement meeting room, an Australian man attired in
turban, orange gown and white pants sat at a table. Tall and thin, with a
bony nose, and long flowing red hair, he appeared to be in his late thirties.
There were only four of us there, and we placed our folding chairs in a
small circle. The monk smiled, enjoying the effect his exotic appearance
had on us. He closed his eyes for a few moments. Then he began to
speak. "Thanks for coming. My name is Acharya Anainjana Brahmacarya.
As that's quite a mouthful, you can call me Dada A."

Wasting no time, he plunged into his topic. "In yoga, we try to
gain a mental equilibrium, so that we can focus on God. What does this
mean, exactly? Just sitting around thinking about God? Just saying, 'God,
God, God?' Of course not." He looked at each of us. "It involves a
transformation, a shift in consciousness, so that you become different.
The heart overflows, the mind is at peace."

I had never really doubted whether some greater presence
existed. The question for me was what to do about it. I was not, in
walking out of the church a few years earlier, declaring that God was
dead. The substance of relating to God, the relationship that I was led

into as a Preacher's Kid, was entrenched in me. I realized that it simply needed shaping. *Deepening.*

After the talk I remained in my chair until the others had left the room. Dada packed up his things, turned to me and smiled, and then asked the question that would change my life, "So, do you want to learn meditation?"

"Sure, I think I do."

"What you want is spiritual experience, not faith." ⟵ *what it is I want*

I stared at him. That *was* really what I was after, through all the chaotic explorations of the past few years. "Yes, I guess that's right."

I agreed to meet him the next day to "take initiation." He arrived at Helios House and I showed him around. Then he went to wash up, splashing water on his face, arms and legs, and instructing me to do the same.

Initiation, he said, was a spiritual transmission by which the aspirant's physical, mental and spiritual condition was changed through a transfer of energy. Initiation created a link with the Guru, as the embodiment of truth.

"I am not the guru," Dada said. "But there is one who initiates you through me."

I didn't grasp much of this at the time. It was only later as I prepared to go to Calcutta to see Baba that it began to make more sense. But I was impressed with this strange man, his dedication to a higher calling, as well as his light-hearted presence.

We sat together in my upper room and he initiated me into the practice of Tantric yoga meditation. I took an oath—something about always doing good to others. And I agreed to give the practice a chance, to sit twice a day for the next two weeks, and, after Dada returned from his travels, to talk with him about how it had gone.

The next day, I sat alone beneath an open window, withdrawing from the usual dramas of the housing co-op. And after some time of breathing and focusing, something happened. My mind felt as if it were slowly expanding, a cloud in the sky, growing larger and larger. Thoughts—of pain, obligation, whimsy, of *lunch*—which usually preoccupied me, slid unceremoniously away.

In a few months I would meet the nun who would invite me to come to Bangkok. Looking back it seems as if these series of events were funneling me toward one goal. Things I hadn't understood before would become clearer, strands weaving together, disparate snatches of melody merging into one song. But of course I didn't see this yet.

For now, sitting in my room at Helios, surrounded by my books, my records, my revolutionary posters, I drifted in and out of a quiet mental oasis. I found my mind observing itself, calm and solid, large and full. Stillness gripped me.

And it was good.

Chapter Nine

These days I awoke early in Thailand, the dawn a whisper of color on the horizon. Within the portal between darkness and the first hint of morning, the room was often still, a stillness that seemed a defined presence, not an absence. My mind was also still. The few belongings I'd carried across the Pacific in my backpack stood in the corner. But these things did not stir a longing for home. Like the slow change of light as night gave way before a tropical dawn, my past also seemed slowly to be dimming, while something else took shape in its place.

"Listen. This is one of my favorite Baba stories."

At breakfast a monk visiting from Calcutta peered at those of us sitting around the newspaper tablecloth, and he launched into a tale. It was a story not about Anandamurti's philosophical insights, or intellectual prowess, or even organizational genius. This story tapped Baba's spiritual power, plain and simple.

A man named Bindeshvari, an early devotee, was attending a convocation with Baba. Succumbing to illness, he actually keeled over and died right then and there. While everyone else was panicking, Baba noted that although the man was technically dead, the vital airs had not completely left the body. Using his healing powers, the story went, he resurrected the man, even after doctors had declared him deceased. There ensued pandemonium, tears of joy, shocked disbelief. And afterwards, Bindeshvari was a changed man, as if somehow Baba had injected him with a new energy. He would fall into *samadhi*—a state of meditative absorption—whenever he saw Baba, and he himself developed an ability to transport other people into ecstasy simply by touching their foreheads.

This story touched something in us. The monks uttered little sighs, or *Hmmms*, gazing into the middle distance in dreamy satisfaction as it concluded. I also enjoyed it, though perhaps not as much as these men who had spent time with Baba.

In the year or so before coming abroad, stories of mystics and saints had seized my imagination like prairie grass shooting out runners in a fertile plain. I'd pored over books from various traditions, searching for transcendence. The tales I read inspired me, but they were often symbolic or filtered through many (sometimes thousands) years of collective imagining. Suddenly I was being offered a steady diet of stories about a living, breathing man who seemed plugged into the Cosmic Grid completely, and they boggled my mind.

As often happened, the story triggered a narrative chain reaction. "Here's another one."

Baba was traveling by train between the Indian cities of Delhi and Ranchi. The train was scheduled to stop at a certain town along the way, and a poor man, having heard that Baba would be passing by, decided to walk the 35 kilometers from his village to see his teacher at this station. The man rose early, and his elderly mother, who also longed to see Baba but couldn't walk so far, gave him a pot of yogurt to carry as a gift. The man then hurried along his route, but had not reached the town by the time the train was to leave.

Mysteriously, though, the train was delayed at this station for an hour and a half, for no reason that the engineer or anyone else could fathom. It simply would not move. The man finally arrived, exhausted, and threw himself at Baba's feet on the platform. Baba pulled him up and stroked his tear-stained cheeks, asking him how he was.

"And, do you have some yogurt for me?"

"Oh!" He had put the pot down on a bench before running to greet Baba. The man then presented the gift to Baba, who smiled and conversed with him, then gave the man's cheek one last caress, and got back on the train. Everyone reboarded, and the train for some equally mysterious reason was able to move again.

"Or this one." The dada brushed some papaya seeds into a plastic bag, crumpled up the newspaper tablecloth and smiled at me.

Sitting near Baba a man thought to himself, "Is it true that Baba knows my thoughts all the time? If it is, he will look at me now!" Baba glanced over at him.

This sequence was repeated three times, Baba glancing over at the man at precisely the moment he thought in this way. Each time the person figured it was a fluke and resolved to test Baba once again.

Finally, exasperated, Baba turned to the man and said, "Why are you thinking like this?"

I loved these stories. I heard a lot of them in Bangkok. The people who told them were generally intelligent, often with a healthy sense of humor and common sense. I tended to trust them. And they offered insight into a world I wanted to be part of.

Yet these tales were also floating me into unknown waters, reframing as they did the little matter of the commonly accepted structure of reality. Spiritual masters, especially this one, inhabited a world in which the physical laws of the universe were mutable. How was this possible?

Maybe such bending of the rules did follow an internal logic—it made sense according to spiritual philosophy, in which everything was connected. Meditation was about expanding your consciousness, and the more it expanded the more you became in tune with other minds, up to the state of God-realization. I'd read that many realized masters were known for their miraculous powers. This could explain Baba's omniscience.

In Austin I'd read *The Autobiography of a Yogi*, a sweet little book in which the author Swami Yogananda described his first meetings with his guru. From this I'd been able to parse something of the guru's role. As far as I could understand, it was to point the way to the divine presence. But also to radiate a love of such intensity that the aspirant got a taste of what God was really like. The physical guru was not God, but God's grace might be manifested through such evolved beings. The flame of one lamp lights up countless lamps. So I was not taken completely by surprise by these stories about Baba as an all-knowing, all-loving teacher.

Still, as I began to get caught up in the heady buzz surrounding him, I tried to remain open-minded. I'd also read the philosopher Krishnamurti, who at a young age had been declared the new messiah by zealous followers, but who eventually turned his back on all of that. After this he inveighed against the need to follow anyone at all. Humans did not come to truth through any guru, any master, any method, but only through the pure, rational search for it, he said. I didn't entirely buy this, though I admired his forthrightness.

Stories I'd read about the corruption or quackery of some gurus also made me cautious. I'd been around enough conservatively religious-minded folks in Texas to see that the devout often look for confirming evidence in what they wish to believe, and ignoring whatever discounts it.

Conversely I knew many young people who declined to get involved in any kind of organized religious experience, or make any communal commitment. They didn't trust the compromises required to belong to a group, rightly suspicious of organized religion's history. But though I shared some of these concerns, such a reluctance seemed a baby and bathwater calculation.

I have to say I had a good feeling about things. This was due in part, I think, to the people I admired who spoke so highly of Baba, partly to the slowly transformative power of the meditation practices, and partly to the ideals of service and universalism Baba espoused.

Plus, I was a sucker for the stories.

If, as now seemed increasingly likely, I was going to India myself, I wanted to have some further grounding. And so I decided to gather information about Baba.

Here was the picture I pieced together: He was born to Bengali parents in 1921 in Jamalpur, Bihar, in the northeastern part of India. His father was a civil servant. His birthday was the same as the Buddha's 2500 years earlier (an auspicious day). He was given the name Prabhat Ranjan Sarkar, a name suggestive of the color of the rising sun.

When he was a boy, he had often been seen wandering among the forested hills near his home, spending hours at a stretch alone, often in meditation. At age seven, the story goes, his elder sister rebuked him for spending so much time alone and not learning anything. Calmly he reached for a pad and pen, and surprised her by writing his name in the scripts of seven different languages. Clearly, he was an unusual child.

In his teenage years he's said to have regularly given away whatever money he had to the needy. He had a reputation for possessing certain psychic abilities and for being able to offer practical advice to people in trouble, and many people in his town availed themselves of his capacity to answer questions, whether about locating lost relatives or dealing with health crises.

At some point, the young man had a realization, apparently, about his own calling. He himself had no guru, no spiritual teacher, but if the claims can be believed, he was born into this world with a deep understanding of and connection to divine energy.

Sarkar moved to Calcutta to attend college where his calling became clearer. One story especially struck a chord with me. One evening while he was sitting alone on the banks of the Hooghly River in a desolate area outside the city, a criminal crept up, intent on mischief. I imagine the man approaching from behind, a dagger clutched in a sweaty palm. Baba spoke to him without turning around.

"You can have whatever I have, Kalicharan," he said, addressing the man by name. "But you can't go on living the way you are."

The thief was taken aback. No one had ever spoken to him like this. In fact, no one had paid him much attention at all, apart from the fear he inspired in his victims. After further conversation, Kalicharan accepted Baba as his master, learned sadhana, and agreed to leave his life of crime. This was Baba's first initiation as a teacher, and after this he began to teach meditation to many others, though he required a commitment to a high standard of ethical conduct from anyone who wanted to learn.

In Calcutta his tremendous intellect also came into sharp focus; he began corresponding with a number of well-known political figures, such as Subhas Chandra Bose, Bengal's preeminent freedom fighter against British imperialism, and radical humanist M. N. Roy, about the question of wartime cooperation with the British. Later, he corresponded with the president of a leading party about the demarcation of borders related to the upcoming partition of India and Pakistan. Sarkar had been critical of partition, and thought the nation could have been saved with the proper approach. This was when he first came to the attention of Jawaharlal Nehru, soon to be India's first prime minister, who reportedly told his security services to keep an eye on this man, P. R. Sarkar.

Baba was a remarkable figure. Yet for many years he remained tucked away into the fold of a seemingly ordinary life, a diamond in a vein of coal. After college he worked as an accountant in the vast Indian National Railway bureaucracy. He lived in Bihar state, a lawless, Wild West kind of place. His co-workers say he was extremely disciplined in his work habits and had no tolerance for bribery. In those early days he had only a few spiritual followers. They would sit with him in a special place after work, "the tiger's grave" outside of Jamalpur, where he performed demonstrations related to the existence of *kundalini, cakras,* and *samadhi.* It's said he healed people's illnesses, answered their questions, or revealed information about their past (though he generally discouraged people from pursuing knowledge of past lives, claiming such knowledge was distracting). All this he did in a humble, gracious, and firm manner.

Like threads woven into a colorful skein, there grew around him a circle of disciples. In 1955, leaving his work with the railways, he founded the organization I was now becoming a part of, Ananda Marga Pracaraka Samgha, "the Association for the Propagation of the Ideals of the Path of Bliss." It was called Ananda Marga for short (and I shorthand it even further as AM). In the years following, this organization grew by the thousands, the tens of thousands, and then the hundreds of thousands. Members of AM were known as "margiis." Opening free schools and clinics across India, they became active in disaster relief, expanding the organization first in Bihar and Bengal, then into other parts of India, and eventually all around the world.

Baba laid out what he expected of his followers in a concise spiritual regimen that he called "the sixteen points." These covered practices such as yoga asanas, the lessons of Tantra sadhana, and practical advice on food, bathing, health, etc. They also included a commitment to the ethical code of Yama and Niyama, ten points such as non-stealing, truthfulness, cleanliness, non-accumulation, and mental contentment. (His interpretation of *ahimsa*, or non-harming, did not preclude the use of force to protect the innocent). Those who adhered to these points, Baba intimated, would find their lives transformed and would move with speed toward their spiritual goal. I'd begun to learn about and embrace these points since coming to Asia, and had found them very useful.

He worked long hours and demanded as much of his followers. "Find satisfaction in meditation and right relationship," he instructed. "Don't fritter away your energy with bad habits or the pursuit of wealth, which in the end bring little happiness." Tranquil and self-controlled, he was said to be able to raise his own kundalini and that of others as well. The awakening of this spiritual energy said to lie dormant in the base of the human spine was a likely explanation for the blissful states that disciples often experienced in his presence. From all reports, his energy seemed boundless, his ideas and projects unending. Baba's writings would eventually include an encyclopedia on the Bengali language, and over 200 books containing essays on agriculture, ethics, health and natural medical treatment, the arts, crime and punishment.

On most Sunday afternoons he gave lectures at his home to an ever-growing number of people, including many international visitors. In these weekly gatherings one of his main themes was the cultivation of the inner life.

"Train yourself in the ideal of the lily," he wrote, "which blossoms in the mud and has to keep itself engaged in the struggle for existence day in and day out...and yet it does not forget the moon above. It seems a most ordinary flower. Still this most ordinary little flower has a romantic tie with the great moon..."

Listening to his voice on a tape which I came across, I heard him say, "Be God-loving, not God-fearing." His voice was mellifluous, and he stretched out his vowels as if to emphasize the importance of what he was saying. "Do not say you are a sinner. You are the sons or daughters of the Cosmic Father."

What really interested me was that in the mid-1960's, Sarkar began advancing a socio-economic gospel of equitable wealth distribution and democratic, decentralized control of the economy. These ideas, spelled out in his Progressive Utilization Theory, or PROUT, signaled a radical stepping away from the traditional domain of Indian gurus, who tended not to focus on social or economic matters. Many people embraced these ideas and in cities, towns, and villages across eastern India, graffiti— "PROUT: the need of the hour!" or "Rational Distribution of Resources!"—began to appear.

I learned that Sarkar was strong in his critiques of both capitalism and communism. West Bengal's Marxist government sought to discredit him, as I understood it, because his service projects drew people away from the politicized commitments that the Marxists wanted to instill in their own followers. India's central government was also, apparently, getting nervous about this galvanizing figure.

In the early 70's in India, the fires of revolution smoldered. Social and economic inequities were coming under increasing criticism from a radicalized youth population. Several times the government attempted to suppress Sarkar, though with little success. Stresses were appearing as well within his organization, which now claimed upwards of several million members.

As happens sometimes in the lives of great people, controversy flared. The Indian government claimed that a power clash between monks within Ananda Marga led to violence and that several people were killed. Spokespersons for the organization said it was a setup. Sarkar was charged with conspiracy to murder, a charge most people who've reviewed the case consider trumped up. Soon after this, reacting to a volatile political situation, Prime Minister Indira Gandhi swept the political landscape starkly clean with imposition of martial law. All opposition leaders were jailed.

Prabhat Sarkar spent seven years in jail, yet continued to direct the operations of AM from there. Most margiis had gone underground or faced imprisonment and torture. I was shocked to learn that after Sarkar's first two years in prison, the Central Intelligence Bureau tried to poison him. He survived this assassination attempt, and though greatly weakened, he fasted, as protest, on two cups of liquid a day for the next five years. If I understood it correctly, the feat was representative of a tremendous spiritual power—the ability to draw sustenance from the vital energy in the air around him.

In 1977, heeding an outcry by international human rights groups like Amnesty International and by legal scholars about the lack of judicial process Sarkar had been afforded, the new post-Indira government cleared him of all charges and released him from prison. It was a red-letter day in the history of Ananda Marga. After a celebration, he returned to his work of writing, organizing and meeting with spiritual aspirants.

Learning this history, I was inspired by the details of this man's life. I was also, I admit, concerned about the controversial bits. Given his criticism of powerful elements in society, it made sense that he had been persecuted, and perhaps it meant that his ideas and movements were making a mark. It was also possible, of course, that some of Sarkar's followers had gotten mixed up in acts of violence, perhaps reacting to government provocation. Exactly what had happened during that period was not clear, and not easy to get information about. For now, the organization's focus was very much on the work of the moment.

But the scope of Sarkar's teachings, his actions, and the extraordinary effects he had on all of these people, suggested to me that he was worth knowing. His *story* compelled me. There was much that was still mysterious about him. It was a mystery I wanted to solve.

PART TWO — CALCUTTA

Chapter Ten

I was traveling with an American monk in his late 20's named Dada Prahlad, a jovial guy who didn't sweat the little things.

I was, finally, in India.

Our hotel in Delhi was a molting colonial house with chunks of mortar occasionally slipping from the outer walls and crashing into the dusty courtyard. Exhausted by the rigors of the flight from Bangkok, we'd slept late. I was awakened around noon by a disturbance in the street four stories below. Prying the window open I stuck my head out. A couple of ragtag kids had a little vaudeville act going on down below with a live monkey.

As the boy beat the tambourine, the girl jerked her limbs around like a slam-dancer, cavorting with the monkey, which was wearing a tattered red skirt and a tasseled hat. When they were done, they looked up to my window, hoping I would throw down some rupees for their trouble. How could I refuse such a welcome?

From Delhi we caught a train, momentum hurtling us toward our final destination of Calcutta. Though to use the term "hurtling" in conjunction with Indian trains was pushing things. The Giitanjali Express made its Delhi-Calcutta run in just under a day and a night.

On the train, uniformed stewards served tasty vegetarian food, and we were chilled by the heavy air conditioning, a counterpoint to the heat pressing down outside like a giant mitt. We bustled through Agra and in the middle distance could see the Taj Mahal, monument to eternal love. The Indians ignored it, but Prahlad and I crowded close to the barred windows. Even from this distance the elaborate scale of the palace was remarkable, the giant domed roof towering over reflecting pools. Later we passed Varanasi, where crowds of orthodox Hindus flocked to take purifying dips in the Ganges. In India the landmarks seemed as often spiritual as physical: Mount Rushmores of devotion, Monticellos of realization.

"India is not some mystical, ancient land of wisdom. It's a place like any other," an anthropology professor once told me. Fair enough. And yet I wanted to believe that something special could happen here. Thomas Merton, arriving in India, had experienced an awakening. "I know and have seen what I was obscurely looking for," he wrote in his Asian diaries. Epiphanies, openings, awakenings, *were* possible, I told myself.

I was comforted by the possibility of "holy human beings" treading in the muck of this world. One of the great exemplars of such devotion was Caetanya Mahaprabhu. Born in 1486, his fits of divine madness acted as a model for succeeding generations of devotees. Dancing in the street like a drunkard, he let all practical concern slip away from him like dross, stepping deeper and deeper into a river of ecstasy. Without love, rituals are useless, he intimated. Under Caetanya's influence, eastern India was swept by a passion for *kiirtan* chanting, ecstasy seizing everyone regardless of social class.

We chugged past a smoky village of some twenty mud-brick houses. A turbaned peasant walked in the field, swatting his bull with a tree branch as he escorted it home for the evening. Children splashed in a shallow pond, and the smoke of a dozen cooking fires wreathed the tops of the pipal trees casting a shade over the village.

"Tell me a story, Dada."

My companion looked at me and smiled. He thought for a moment. "True story. There once was a margii who came from a small, isolated island in the south Pacific to see Baba. A new devotee. He didn't know much about the organization, didn't even speak English, and yet he had some feeling for Baba."

"When he arrived in Calcutta, he had an opportunity for personal contact—just he and Baba alone. And guess what Baba did? I'll tell you. He spoke for a long time to this man in his native tongue, some obscure Polynesian language that only people from that island group speak! The man was beaming from ear to ear when he came out of the room."

Prahlad settled back with a sigh. "Yup," he said. "There's nobody like Baba."

I settled back, too. Prahlad had probably not been that different from me when he'd been a student back in the U. S. But he'd committed to monk's vows, and now was living a very different life. As for me, I was still unsure of my place in the world. Maybe Baba was someone who could reveal to me the unconscious impulses that drove me, often in the wrong direction. Perhaps he could lift me out of myself, show me the limitations of my own ego, as well as a vision of what I might become.

I didn't know if my earlier darkness and my pressing need to get away from the States were part of my karma, a set of experiences I'd needed to go through in order to arrive at this space and time. But as I looked out the window at the dusty countryside, trying to picture Caetanya's time, and trying to imagine meeting a modern-day guru, I sensed something. I felt I was being called. Someone was calling me.

Around ten o'clock in the morning we pulled into Calcutta's Howrah Station. Cal, I later heard the city called. Into Cal poured the great British train lines and Indian Air lines as well as the poleboats, with their boatmen yodeling songs of the Gangetic plains. Above Cal, the smog of thousands of taxis and millions of cookfires drifted. Through Cal shot a new subway line, fractured because of poor workmanship and heavy rains soon after its inception.

Because of Cal, because of who was in Cal, I came. And in spite of Cal, I would stay.

Howrah was bedlam, a great jostling of bodies across the sweeping central space, bodies hugging twine-tied bundles and bags, bodies asleep in rows on the concrete floor waiting for a late train, a crush of bodies log-jammed at the rickety exit stiles. And outside, a barrage of bodies, porters, taxi drivers, money changers, dope peddlers and hotel agents pestering the traveler, especially the foreign traveler, as he made his way into the city.

We avoided these and caught a local bus. It inched along under the steel suspension cables of Howrah Bridge, jockeying for position with hundreds of Ambassador cars and Tata trucks blaring their horns, belching black smoke, while rickshaws pulled by barefoot, bare-chested men in *lungis* wove in and out of the traffic. Then it was down into the twisting lanes and thoroughfares of the city, past stately British-era monuments and mausoleums. Down the side streets lay endless shops, typists sitting on wooden crates pecking out letters for the illiterate, vendors selling cigarettes, pots and pans, or fruits and vegetables out of tiny cupboards attached to the buildings.

Through the louvered windows of the houses I could see lazily revolving ceiling fans, while on the sidewalk men carrying unopened umbrellas ambled by, shawls spread around their shoulders, ignoring the skeletal street dogs which wavered in their way.

As Baba was a Bengali, I'd taken an interest in the region and tried to read what I could about it. In the 1960's, the rise of a revolutionary Marxist terrorism had gripped Bengal, followed by massive government repression. Bengal was thrown into further turmoil during Bangladesh's war with Pakistan as a heavy influx of refugees poured into the state. All of this prepared the way for the emergence of the Communist government that ruled in the 1980's. The American embassy now sat forlornly on an avenue that had, in a sly political barb, been renamed Ho Chi Minh Street. I imagined the American ambassador sighing each morning as he opened each letter addressed to the U. S. embassy, care of Uncle Ho.

Prahlad had to get off downtown to do an errand, and so left me with instructions for finding my stop alone. On a narrow residential street lined with two-story pale brick houses behind gates, I found the address, and as I was entering the building, a monk dressed in orange hurried out. Yes, this was the right place. The man looked me over, was about to move on, and then stopped. He pulled me aside. "May I have 100 rupees?" What was this? I dug in my pocket and forked over a 100-rupee note. The dada thanked me and continued out the gate.

Just then, another monk opened the door and welcomed me into the house.

"Did he ask you for money?" this second man asked. "Scoundrel. We have a lot of work to do, and the pressure for money gets to be too much sometimes."

It did seem a strange welcome. Yet there was no denying that Westerners visiting India often had more money than locals. And when I saw the conditions in which some of the Indian monks and nuns labored, I became more willing to share what I had. There'd always been something of the spendthrift about me. Recently, I had tried to relax this tendency.

The monk invited me to rest for a while. When he was done with his work he accompanied me to Tiljala, a poor neighborhood on the outskirts of Calcutta. Here AM's global headquarters were housed in two massive five-story buildings, one for men and another for women, within two sprawling compounds. Around the outer walls stood smaller buildings—a dusty shop selling fruit and a few yellowing stationary supplies, a communal kitchen, a small post office. A couple of cows loitered on the grass. Behind the main building stood a green stucco house where Baba stayed when he came to Tiljala.

Dada led me up the concrete steps to the fourth floor of the men's jagrti. An open elevator shaft fronted the staircase, and our conversation echoed down the hole. Piles of bricks lay in corners. The building was only a few years old, and seemed oddly unfinished.

The room to which I was shown was large, opening onto a balcony overlooking the campus. It was reserved for people coming from Southeast Asia, though no one seemed to be there at the moment. I unpacked a little and organized my things. Through the grill above the door to the attached bathroom floated the cadences of a Sanskrit chant sung in a deep bass voice. Someone *was* here.

An Indian man stepped out of the bathroom, dripping slightly, a towel around his midsection. "Do you know this mantra?" he asked me. "I pay respect to the sages who came before me." He toweled himself dry as he spoke.

"The act of offering is sacred, that which is offered is sacred, the One to whom it is offered, ahhh, is sacred, the one doing the offering is sacred. Those who, ahhh, relinquish their ego in the act, merge with God when the act is done. It is a beautiful idea." So it was.

I bathed, then sat for meditation. Afterwards I climbed to the roof to check things out. Steel rebar jutted from the concrete along the retaining wall. The smoky sprawl of the suburbs of Calcutta lay on one side, and on the other, open country, rutted bicycle paths linking our village with outlying houses.

Two young Indian monks strolled the perimeter of the roof, holding hands. Several other people gathered on a canvas tarp, enjoying the coolness of the early evening. They munched on what looked like puffed rice and chunks of dried molasses.

A tall Indian sitting on one of the tarps beckoned. "Won't you join us? Where are you from, my dear?"

I sat down on the edge of their group. "Ummm, Bangkok," I said. "I mean I live there now, but I'm..."

They laughed. "You don't look like someone from Thailand."

"I'm American."

"Anyway, it doesn't matter. In the end, we're all from the same place, no?"

Someone unveiled a special snack.

"Aha—great minds think alike," one of the monks laughed. "You see, we really are a universal mission. Everyone likes this white chocolate."

Baba's house in Lake Gardens, a suburb of southern Calcutta, was a rickshaw and two bus rides away from Tiljala. I made the trip with an Australian named Jayanta who had lived in Calcutta for some years and who was writing a book about Baba's economic ideas. We rode past shops, tattered cinema posters plastered over patched mortar walls with "Long Live CPI Marxist" slogans stenciled on them, and blocks of crumbling houses.

"Look at this," Jayanta said. "There's no need for people to live in these conditions. If the Marxists were serious about change, they'd address the housing problem. Crack down on the outflow of capital from the state. Stimulate local economic projects."

I listened with interest, but soon we were arriving at the sweet shop which marked the beginning of the Lake Gardens neighborhood, and so my attention turned to other things. We walked the two streets to Baba's place. The houses were tightly packed, although Baba's house had a small garden surrounding it. People were everywhere—Indians, Africans, Europeans, North and South Americans, men, women, and children, milling about in the street, laughing, chatting. The day was warm, and the vendor of coconut water was making a fortune.

But where was the person I had come to see? Each afternoon, apparently, Baba was driven to a nearby park in order to walk around the lake. When he returned he would take his seat in a cane chair in the driveway of his home and meet with devotees.

Jayanta suggested I find a good place to stand and ducked inside the gate. I watched him press his way through the crowd. Not quite ready to go in, I strode in the street for a while. Anxiety bubbled below the surface of my excitement.

Suddenly a car turned the corner 100 yards away, and a cry went up from the crowd. "He's coming, he's coming!" People scrambled to get a good spot, and I was swept along in the rush. The gates to the driveway swung open and a clean-looking Indian sedan turned in. I could barely see the back of a balding head in the back seat. The driver turned off the engine, but it seemed to be taking forever for anyone to get out. My heart pounded.

Then a short older man stepped slowly from the car and held his hands together in the traditional greeting of "Namaskar," taking pains to acknowledge everyone present. He was immaculately dressed in white *kurta* and *dhoti*, the long shirt and wraparound garb of a Bengali gentleman, a silver pen clipped in his shirt pocket. A sense of great dignity radiated from him, yet he was smiling and amiable, chatting in Bengali with several of the Indians standing nearby.

I knew he was around 60, but his face seemed younger and playful. Clean-shaven, he wore old-fashioned black-framed eyeglasses, the kind widely available in India, hooked over his large and elongated ears, framing a smooth brown face. He shuffled over to sit in a chair beneath a statue of poet Rabindranath Tagore. Everyone moved to stand near him, and someone began to sing, one of the several thousand songs Baba had composed to date. Baba tilted his head and listened, then nodded and smiled.

"Do you like this song?" he asked after it was over. He had an unusual way of speaking, rather formal. "This song is a *ghazal*. The melody is Persian in origin."

His every gesture seemed measured, as if what he had to say carried great weight. I also liked his good humor.

But was this all?

I'd been in Cal now for a few days, settling into a daily routine, enjoying the meals and the companionship. I'd seen Baba twice at Lake Gardens, watched everyone fall all over themselves to be near him, but to tell the truth, I didn't feel much of anything. He seemed an intelligent and sweet, but rather ordinary, old man.

Still, something drew me to make the hour-long journey to his house every day. Perhaps it was a fascination with the workings of the organization, or a fondness for Baba's songs. I loved those songs. Perhaps it was the peaceful quiet of the garden outside Baba's house, or the company of so many kind, progressive people. Or perhaps it was something else, a kind of inchoate longing, as if I felt something special could happen, if only I gave it time.

One day, I sat on the stoop of the neighbors' house, moving respectfully out of the way when they returned from the market. As usual, the area in front of Baba's house was completely packed; my chances of getting close to him there were slim. So when his car arrived I decided to position myself to the side, next to the gate. An Indian man began to warble one of the songs in classical style, and the crowd followed in call and response mode. Everyone was singing earnestly, but I found myself just drifting. The song went on. The sun bore down on the back of my neck. Then, for seemingly no reason, Baba turned his head and glanced at me, standing off to the side.

What happened next is difficult to explain. A Sanskrit word— *darshan*—describes the process by which an exchange takes place through the medium of the eyes, especially between master and disciple. The word literally means "to see," but the connotation in this instance is not of passive viewing, but rather of energetic exchange.

At this tender glance from him my mind soared. It was as if Baba looked straight into my soul and turned up its temperature. I almost had the sensation that little lightning bolts passed between our eyes. I felt real joy, as the usual background roar of worry and fear dropped away completely.

I'd always craved attention and always felt an outsider, wanting people to see me, who I really was. With one glance, Baba gave me that which I needed. *It's all OK*, his smile seemed to say. *Nothing will hurt you, can hurt you. You don't have to try so hard. This state you're experiencing now is what it's really all about.*

It's not that I *believed* in Baba, wraping my cognitive faculties around what I thought was the truth. Critical judgment didn't go out the window, but my analytical mind no longer held primacy, as my consciousness settled into a clarity deep and still as a heavy snow on pine boughs. There was no question of doubt or belief. Rather I had an experience. And this, it seemed, was the profound benefit of contact with a Tantric guru, someone who had the ability to radiate spiritual power, a reflection of divine love.

I didn't know it then, but this moment would stick with me, imprinted on my memory. Through whatever twists and turns my life would take, it would remain, steadfast, and sustaining.

The look lasted for only a few seconds. Then Baba turned and the world began spinning again. I didn't want to talk to anyone and wandered off down the street to be alone. I wanted only to hold on to this sweetness for as long as possible, to hoard it, store it, and flow away into a new realm on the waves generated by that indescribable compassionate gaze.

Chapter Eleven

When I was little, maybe six years old, I used to borrow a large hand mirror from my mother's dresser. If I held it face up and parallel to the floor, I could see the ceiling of our El Paso house reflected in the glass. Focusing intently on this out-of-the-way reality, I would walk around the interior of the house, pretending I was walking on that ceiling.

The floor plan allowed me to move in a large circle, passing through each room: high-stepping over the tops of doorframes, maneuvering around light fixtures, inspecting heating ducts, inching along the wider ledges that separated rooms. I was traveling through a neglected, unfamiliar terrain, in defiance of gravity. It was great fun. I pretended that this was how people moved in China, though I was pretty sure that wasn't true.

Tilting the mirror slightly I could see my parents' religious art on the walls flip-flopped, the folded hands of the devout pointed toward the earth. Guided by the light waves bouncing off the glass, I experienced a little epiphany: our everyday existence was not the only reality. I had to move my body in a new way, tentatively, gingerly, in order to keep pace with this shift, this different perspective my mind had perceived. It was a radical new perception—moving through a world turned upside down.

Now, in India, too, I was moving through a different world, an upside-down world, except that what I was experiencing wasn't due to any trick of mirrors. It was as if I'd begun to glimpse a hidden reality, the reflection of light underlying our reality focused, like the sun's rays through a magnifying glass, into my mind and heart, the obscure layers of our complicated existence beginning to be laid clean, as one wave of extraordinary experience after another lapped up on my thirsty shore.

I was far from my previous life, and it was time to stop dwelling in that past.

CHAPTER TWELVE

Baba presided over a series of gatherings every few months. Tens of thousands of people attended these gatherings which were known as Great Circles of Dharma—Dharma Maha Cakras or DMCs. The next one was going to be held soon, in Tatanagar, a city several hundred miles to the west of Calcutta. Inspired by my brief encounters with this man, I decided to go.

The Tatanagar stop was part of a multi-leg journey, a tour of Northeast India during which Baba lectured on the historical and cultural significance of each city he passed through. He traveled from Lumbini, birthplace of the Buddha, to the area that gave birth to the Nath movement of mystics. He also visited the gravesite of Kabir, great mystic beloved of both Hindus and Muslims. His insights from that tour were collected in a book.

I'd heard that DMCs were special. The program lasted for three days, and featured music and dramatic presentations the first two nights, and organizational meetings during the day. On the final night Baba generally gave a lecture, and then he blessed the crowd with a bestowal of spiritual energy, employing something called the *varabhaya mudra*.

Mudras, I knew, were meaningful hand gestures—I thought of those iconographic representations of the Buddha I'd seen with hand extended in blessing. In fact, religious figures throughout history had appeared in such forms. That energy might be dispensed through such gestures was something I hadn't known.

The big tent was packed that night in Tatanagar. After wandering around outside for a while and checking out the booths selling books, incense and clothes, I squeezed into the tent and sat in the middle of the crowd. The stage was decorated with large papier-mache guitars and tabla drums. A sea of orange uniforms bobbed near the front of the tent. Next to me a family of farmers sprawled on a blanket, sharing a snack from a tattered bag. Across the crowd I spotted an education professor I'd met in Bangkok. We shared a smile.

A cry went up and all eyes turned toward the entrance behind the stage. Walking slowly, carrying his cane, dressed in a white *kurta* and beige *punjabi*, Baba entered. He greeted the crowd and walked to his seat. I found I couldn't take my eyes off him.

The program began. Immediately I was knocked clean out of any state of ordinariness as thirty men—fiery torches in one hand, skulls in the other—leapt into the air. They began the rhythmic jumping of *Tandava*, the dance of Shiva in his *Nataraja* form, an exercise that had been resurrected by Baba. It was a bold and symbolic dance, representing the eternal struggle between opposing forces. Death on one hand and the life force on the other. The overcoming of lethargy through energetic effort. *Eros*, perhaps, and *thanatos*. A recognition of mortality tied to a sense of transcendence.

The men leaped again and again, their torches blazing, their legs kicking high into the air. It was a strange tantric scene.

Watching, I grew thoughtful. There was in me, I knew, an eagerness to please. Even when I'd rebelled as a teenager, my rebellion was often circumscribed, one eye cocked toward the expectations of those around me. Here in the evocative movements of these dancers I witnessed the demonstration of a calm, manly, vital presence, reminding me that what I wanted most was to develop a sense of inner authority.

The men finished and left the stage. The tent grew silent, save for the fluttering of thousands of paper fans. Baba began to speak.

"Everything moves in this universe; everywhere there is expressed dynamicity. Nothing is static in this universe of ours….It is the duty of each and every human being to see that there remains movement in his or her mental world…" The talk went on for some time.

Near the end he shifted gears. "Let everyone be-e-e happy," he said, with the cadence of a blessing. "Let e-e-everyone see the bright side of everything."

A leap in barometric pressure was taking place inside the tent. I glanced around, noticed people straightening, leaning forward; the whole crowd seemed perched as if on the edge of some revelation.

"Le-e-et everyone be free from ailments of all kinds," Baba continued. "Let no one be forced to undergo a-a-ny difficulties due to pre-e-ssure of circumstance."

Slowly, Baba's hands glided into the position of the mudra. Suddenly, the man in front of me cried out, shuddered, and fell over backwards. Another person began to sob. All around me people were shouting, or trembling, laughing, or weeping.

What the hell was going on? And then I, too, felt something. Cool electricity pulsed through the air. It felt, in that moment, as if Baba was intimating to us the timeless nature of the state of enlightenment, giving us a taste as incentive to deepen our spiritual practices. It was a deep yet subtle feeling that left me feeling refreshed and inspired.

Before that evening, I might have supposed the crowd's response was due to a kind of mass hypnosis, everyone geared up to such a heightened state that when the symbolic moment came, they responded almost unconsciously. And yet this didn't ring true; everyone I spoke with afterwards said they'd felt, as I had, some tangible wave of energy. And each responded, evincing a classic litany of ecstatic religious experience.

Some years later I would see a TV show, a Bill Moyers PBS special about healing and the mind which featured a segment on a *qigong* master who could project energies through his hands, knocking people flat from five feet away without physically touching them. This was the kind of thing I suppose Baba did, except that his energy was infused with a strong spiritual power. It intoxicated you, made you mad for God. No wonder people traveled halfway around the world to receive it. No wonder they committed themselves to work for the AM mission.

As the shock waves subsided, Baba rose and walked slowly toward the exit. A local AM leader held out his hands to make sure Baba didn't trip, and slowly backed down the stairs in this protective, overwhelmed state. And now something else happened. After having given the mudra, it seemed as if Baba's body was composed of thousands of tiny points of light, not one solid substance. He shone, he shimmered, the air around him seemed to dance.

I rubbed my eyes, but the phenomenon of swirling energy persisted. It was as if everything around Baba bobbed up and down on a sea of waves. Maybe it was a result of my own heightened perceptions; maybe Baba was actually radiating this. I honestly don't know. But the scene pierced my soul.

CHAPTER THIRTEEN

Prayer flags snapped in the breeze in front of the tall *stupa*-like Ceylonese temple, semaphoring their invocations to the heavens. Tibetan monks moved through the streets in their deep ochre robes, complementing the bright blues, greens, and reds on the walls of their temple.

From the Bodhgaya bus station I trudged through broken streets and checked in at the rustic Burmese Mission: small cells surrounding a quiet shaded courtyard. The charge was one rupee per night, about five U.S. cents.

I'd returned to Calcutta after the Dharma Maha Cakra and tried to settle back into the daily routine. And yet I'd begun to sense that I needed some space to process what was going on. Things were happening pretty quickly.

I decided to see some sights. Bodhgaya, home of the Bodhi tree, where the Buddha supposedly attained enlightenment 2500 years before, was not far away and a place I wanted to see. It was one of the Four Sacred Buddhist spots, the others being the Buddha's birthplace, the place where he gave his first sermon, and Kasimara, where he died.

I wanted to spend some time alone to try to make sense of things. I still wasn't completely sure that Ananda Marga was my path. Despite the experiences I was having with Baba, on some level the idea of guru still seemed a little crazy. No doubt he was a powerful teacher. But could I let go of my ego and accept him as master?

In India such a relationship had a long pedigree, but in the West it stood against the normative understanding of relationship and authority, in which you grew up, separated from your family, your ego *individuated*; maybe you fell in love and shared your life with another, but you did your best to maintain a sense of individuality and autonomy. That was the norm.

Normal
\
Insane

Balance

On the other hand, what was normal? Normal was just a point on a curve denoting the number of people who subscribed to a certain behavior. Plenty of instances could be noted in which those who were supposedly well-adjusted, when judged against the yardstick of common sense and human feeling, tilted toward the insane, and those who appeared mad held the key to wisdom.

The Buddha's shrine lay on the outskirts of town. Like birds flocking to a feeder, hundreds of pilgrims gathered there—Tibetans, Indians, Westerners. Temples representing the aspirations of each Buddhist country lined the dusty road—spare, pointy-spired Japanese temples; rustic Burmese ones; garish, colorful Chinese temples with red hewn pillars, gongs, and the smoke of incense clogging the air. If a pilgrim walked seven times around the stupa with a sincere mind, he would obtain knowledge of his previous life. At least that's what the placard posted outside the main building said.

Inside the Tibetan temple I was ambushed by a band of boy-monks, six, seven, eight years old, in pint-sized maroon robes, with shaved stubbly scalps. They tailed me around the compound, hoping I'd take their picture, popping their heads out from around corners or at the top of a flight of whitewashed stairs, erupting in giggles.

And then I went to see the Bodhi tree, the huge spreading pipal with multiple trunks like threads in a weave winding around each other. It was several hundred feet of yellow branches and a canopy of dark green leaves. Pilgrims were engaged in a series of prostrations, measuring the circumference of the temple around the tree with their bodies, arms outstretched. There were monks here who'd made pilgrimages of hundreds of miles performed in such prostrations.

Here the Buddha took his stand, or seat, defying convention, ignoring normal patterns of thought, vowing not to move until he was filled with light. He'd been through the ascetic wringer up to this point, exploring a variety of practices. Some of them were so extreme that they'd reduced him to flesh and bones, as he wandered like a matted madman through the villages of northern India. Finally he swung back to the middle of the road, seeking a balanced approach to enlightenment.

In one temple I attended a Western monk's talk on the importance of being free of a false conception of self, of living in the moment, mindfully. We were asked to walk slowly around the temple grounds, one foot in front of the other, rapt in the effortlessness of motion, a courtyard full of snail-paced seekers. As I walked, I did feel peaceful. There was something to learn here. It was good to observe this long tradition with its monks and nuns and family people, all following the teachings of their preceptor.

On the other hand, I knew that Baba, like the Buddha, emphasized living in the present, not being tied to regrets about the past, or expectations of the future. I *was* attracted to the heart-centered nature of AM teachings, the centrality of love or devotion, and service. By comparison, some Buddhism seemed a little dry.

Although Bodhgaya was a spiritual mecca, in the streets a mercenary attitude reigned. On every corner solicitations rang out, "Yah, sir, camera for sale? Flim, sir? You want hashish?" Fortune-seekers swarmed like flies to the honey of foreigners. Each time I stepped outside the walls of the Burmese Mission, I faced a moving wall of human bodies, hands outstretched, repeating the mantra of rupees, surging forward with me as I moved. I admired the hand stenciled T-shirt I saw one traveler wearing which spelled out beneath an encompassing "No!" the list of undesired objects: "Hotel, Rickshaw, Hashish, Change Money." After several days of fending these guys off, I was feeling quite put upon. And conflicted by this anger I felt.

So one morning I walked out of town across the desert toward a small red-clay village in the distance. The oasis lay a half-mile or so to the west, six or seven houses heavily shaded by a copse of banyan trees. It was still early, and the day's heat hadn't yet settled in, but I knew that things would soon be broiling. Some kind of grasshopper leapt in front of me and landed on my thigh. I watched as, with insect stoicism, it rubbed its spindly front legs together and tasted my blue jeans. Its back flashed an intricate green.

Thatched roof houses of woven cane stood on raised foundations of earth, rutted dirt paths connecting the houses. Several villagers stood in the lane, brushing their teeth with twigs plucked from a neem tree. Amidst the sweet pungent smell of frying *luchis*, and the chirruping of cicadas, cookfire smoke settled in wisps over the barrier of trees. I met a young Indian, perhaps 16 years old. He was kind, with an innocent, guileless personality, a welcome antithesis to the touts of Bodhgaya.

I was hot and thirsty and he offered me a bottle of Campa Cola. We chatted for a while and then he invited me to his home, nearby, for an early lunch. We sat and talked while his mother rolled *chapatis* and fried potatoes over an outdoor fire.

"Do you come to see the Buddha, sir?"

"Yes, I wanted to see where the Buddha attained enlightenment."

"He was great soul, sir. Even Hindus, we respect the Buddha."

I smiled at him. "What do you do?"

"I am studying. In the school. Do you want to hear a song?"

Another boy was ushered over to us by a younger brother. The boy's eyes rolled back in their sockets, but his face was sweet. He inched his way forward as he was guided to his seat. Then, grasping a three-stringed lyre, he began to play, and to sing, in a wailing angel's voice. Though his eye cavities were dark, there was light in his face.

"He sings about God, sir."

"I can feel it."

Invocation, incantation, whatever it was, the blind boy evoked some higher presence through the intent focus of his song. We all felt it.

The difficulty of travel in India sometimes gave way to these shining moments of connection and reassurance. You might jostle elbows with poets and mystics and heaven-sent musicians on any corner. My new friend did, in the end, ask for money, telling me that he didn't have enough to pay his school fees this year. I might have flinched at this, but his simplicity seemed to vouchsafe his sincerity, and I gave him 100 rupees. I trusted him, because of his kindness, because of the village, and because of the music. He had made me feel at home.

I walked back across the half-mile of desert with that blind boy's song echoing around my brain.

At the Burmese Mission, I hunkered down in my cell. I was thinking of the stories I'd heard about "holy madness." For example, Simeon, a Christian saint, used to parade the streets of his town, dragging a dead dog behind him on a rope. He slowed in front of shops and cafes, where genteel patrons did double takes. How many of them realized that Simeon was simply giving a nod to the excess baggage everyone toted around? I heard of another reclusive guru who threw stones at any visitors who approached him for advice, perhaps testing their mettle. And didn't one of the great Zen masters attain enlightenment upon hearing the splash of his own turd into the toilet water below? *Crazy wisdom, that.*

What these figures had in common, I decided, was willingness to put the ego in its place. As Joseph Campbell notes, the difference between mystical experience and the psychological crack-up is that the one who cracks is drowning in the same water in which the mystic swims. You had to be prepared for this experience, and you needed help to be prepared.

In this light, was the guru-disciple relationship irrational? Maybe not. If it was about finding someone who could help you cut through the dross, get down into what was real, no matter how unusual it looked from the outside, wasn't that rational? And if not, did it matter? Perhaps the rational mind only went so far.

I had also previously read about the trickster figure. Found in most cultures, the trickster is a mediator between worlds, a wanderer with access to a "way." He points to "opportunity" (from the Greek *poroi*, or portal) and represents looseness in the weave of reality. Perhaps on one level Baba could be seen as a kind of wise trickster, crossing from the cosmic to the quotidian and back again, pointing the way.

What I hadn't yet fully understood was that surrender didn't mean relinquishing autonomy or initiative or any of that. It simply meant discerning, with the help of a competent, evolved teacher, what one's deepest self needed in order to flourish. It meant opening oneself to mystery.

CHAPTER FOURTEEN

After a week in Bodhgaya, I could no longer resist the pull to return to Calcutta, and so I caught a train, eager to see Baba again. Something was tugging at my heart. Perhaps the blind boy had reminded me that when it came to devotional music, Baba was up to something of a different order altogether.

The morning after I got back I took a cab with several Indian acharyas from Tiljala to Lake Gardens. Five of us were crammed in, practically sitting on each other's laps, as happens without a second thought in India. We careened around the wobbly traffic circles of Gariahat and Ballygunge, flying past tailoring kiosks and the Kwality Restaurant. Each time we rounded another perilous curve, we were thrown into each other's arms and someone would cry out, "Oh, ho!" I could tell these guys appreciated a bit of spontaneity. I'd never met several of them before, but as we were all coming from the same place and all headed to the same place, we nursed a budding camaraderie.

Someone launched into a tune. It was the latest song composed by Baba. And suddenly there blazed in my fellow passengers' eyes a new appreciation for the day.

E ki madhurato pabone E ki madokata monone E ki sure sure pakhi gay E ki bhalobasa bhubane.

The melody rose gracefully, and descended, almost like a wave. The song's microtones, fastidiously attempted by these Indian acharyas, made my head buzz. I joined in on the chorus. We hadn't spoken five words to each other before this ride, but once we began singing, we were all fast friends, drinking buddies in the Lord.

"Do you know the translation?" one asked me. I shook my head.

"What is this sweetness on the breeze? What is this mind full of bliss? Why are the birds singing so melodiously? What is this love filling the world?"

He smiled, and I, captivated, smiled back.

And we sailed on through southern Cal, finally tumbling out at Baba's house, where, with a larger crowd, we began to sing again.

Every day, Baba sat in a hard-backed rattan chair in his driveway and invited us to sing back to him his latest compositions. Prasanta Das usually began. A Calcutta devotee with a mesmerizing voice, Prasanta's vowels hummed like a wire in the wind. The air was different after his performance, bringing to mind legends of medieval musicians to whom unusual powers were attributed: their singing of *ragas* was so focused, so intent, that they created bursts of spontaneous combustion, or made the rains come.

Tumi Tumi Tumi, Eso kache aro kache. Please come closer, ever closer.

Some days a Bengali sister elbowed her way through the crowd, asserting her right to sing. She, too, sang beautifully, with leaps and pirouettes of sound, her voice a fountain, a sparkling cascade of rushing water. She scooped up emotion like gems from this stream, panned out of the flow of music and thrown at our feet, raw and unrefined.

Occasionally a group was asked to lead the singing. Not everyone knew the song well; some mumbled in the background while others carried the tune. I got in on this group song-leading once or twice. As the songs were coming fast and furiously, several a day, and a challenge to learn the latest tunes, let alone the lyrics, it was often only later that I learned the meaning of what I sang. The best thing, though, was to have the translation ahead of time, and then the song could work its magic fully.

After we sang, Baba might say, in a voice suffused with love and good humor: "*Acha*, do you like this song? Should we keep it?"

"Yes, Baba."

"*Acha*, it is all by your grace," he would tease. And we melted.

I couldn't get enough of those glorious, haunting tunes, the *Prabhat Samgiit*, or *Songs of the New Dawn* as they were called (a play on Baba's first name, Prabhat). Every one I heard moved me. I was quickly being pulled into a relationship with Baba through these songs. I hadn't been in India long, but I felt connected to what was going on, mainly through this music. Though I might resist some of the discipline, I also saw around me the intoxicated abandon of the devotee who throws the rules out the window in the need to express his love. The many conduct rules, the organizational structure, these things that might occasionally seem controlling or rigid, were oiled, made palatable by what these songs brought forth: ecstatic, spontaneous, non-conforming expressions of devotion.

"Style is a very simple matter," Virginia Woolf wrote. "It is all rhythm. This is very profound, what rhythm is, and goes far deeper than words. A sight, an emotion, creates this wave in the mind, long before it makes words to fit in." Though Woolf was referring to prose, the sentiment certainly holds for music. Faced with the hectic pace of modern life, Baba seemed to be asserting that human beings needed soothing, engaging rhythms of a deep sensibility—we all needed good music, all needed to express ourselves. And did he ever express himself! Between 1983 and 1990 Baba would compose more than 5,000 songs—five thousand and eighteen, to be precise.

Sometimes when hanging out at Lake Gardens during the day I would hear the words "*Gan gan*" (song, song) ring out, and I would watch those in charge of transcribing songs drop what they were doing and rush to Baba's side, notebooks in hand. They were dedicated to the process, first responders. Inspiration might strike when Baba was shaving, or having his meal (or the monks having theirs, for that matter), or when he was engaged in any of the hundred and one projects he was pursuing at the time. This cosmic flow of music erupted at any time, apparently, and could not be stemmed or ignored.

Baba composed in a variety of styles: *ghazal* (Sufi songs), *baul* (the songs of wandering Bengali mystics), folk, and classical Indian tunes. Drawing also on melodies from other cultures such as Persian or Scandinavian, he wrote lyrics, though primarily in Bengali, in other languages, too—Hindi, Urdu, a few in English. You could hear and feel in these songs the mystic's yearning for merger with the infinite, the juicy attraction for God as beloved, as well as a sensibility celebrating the seasons and the natural world.

> *Come, come, come into my heart. With a smile as sweet as honey*
> *Radiating from your rosy feet to your charming face.*
> *I thrill to the sound of your name. I am a canvas for your color.*
> *In your song, everything of mine is reconciled. In contemplation*
> of you, *I lose myself.*
> *Come, come. Come into my heart.*

A few years back, a monk visiting Austin had encouraged the margiis to buy cassettes of these early songs. I hadn't paid much attention. In those days the recordings were tinny, poorly mastered, and no one really knew what they were. That would change as the organization gradually invested in professional recordings, and famous Indian singers became aware of and lined up to sing these marvelous tunes. And the number of songs continues to grow.

I didn't know then as I stood in a driveway of a house in a suburb of Calcutta that this was the beginning of a lifelong fascination for me—a love affair with devotional music, which would eventually lead me to study Bengali, and to begin to help translating *Prabhat Samgiit* (along with other more accomplished translators). This work affected me strongly. My meditation would sometimes become spotty in later days, but sinking into the work of translating these songs, which meant I had to listen and think deeply about their meanings, kept me "in the flow."

I would come to understand what Coleman Barks, who made a name for himself translating Rumi for a Western audience, meant when he said, "The work can involve a kind of emptying out, a surrender. It's also a form of healing, a way to play and praise, and an unfolding friendship with a teacher. Or just say that all these poems are love poems."

Mornings in Tiljala I took a cool shower and folded a blanket on the floor, perhaps pausing to gaze for a few moments out the arched windows of our room at the rice paddies and smoky villages in the distance. Then I pulled from my bag the small notebook containing my ever-expanding collection of songs, with English translations. I was in the habit of singing five or six every day before meditation.

Why did you urge me to leave the house on this rainy day, leaving me without refuge? Why have you created a flood in the dried riverbed of my mind?

I would settle in to singing for up to an hour, and the devotional vibrations deepened like shadows around me. The crowds and dust of Calcutta had a tendency to overwhelm, to singe the tender shoots of my new spiritual aspirations. But sometimes, inside myself, I stumbled across a lush green oasis with irrigating sloughs of crystal-clear water. *Prabhat Samgiit*, to stretch a metaphor, was the music floating across the desert that guided me to that oasis.

In the evening things really flowed. As dusk washed out the rural landscape on the outskirts of the city with pale light, I sensed a change in the world's mood. This was the passing of the *sandhya*, the shift from the rush of day to the deep stillness of night. Correspondingly, I chose a melancholy song.

How many twilights have passed? How many autumn and spring nights? The golden dawn of my life, is it returning again?

At such times bittersweet feelings welled within me. I remembered my teenage angst, the struggles of recent years. And then I felt a rising above these confusions, a connection with something or someone beyond myself. These songs were helping me forge a personal relationship with the divine.

I was, I felt, where I was supposed to be.

One day I visited a Calcutta margii family in their home. There the feeling was again confirmed that an extraordinary energy inhabited the notes and words of this music, that these songs were somehow haunted.

I was invited into the family's spare but comfortable living room. It was an interesting chance for me to connect with people outside the ashram, to get a glimpse into daily life in Calcutta. They were hospitable and wanted to know more about my life in America. After the shortest of meditations—eight minutes—the father asked me to sing. At first shyness held me back. What could I possibly sing? But then I realized I possessed an extraordinary repertoire. By becoming more familiar with Baba's songs, I held a world that would always lift me out of myself.

With a single touch, you could have me. This process of getting acquainted is too drawn out, too lukewarm.

My audience beamed, whether in appreciation of my attempts at Bengali, or simply because of the song's rich sentiment. And suddenly, as so often happened when I sang these songs, I was transported. My mind flared up like a comet, and as soon as I finished singing, I slipped back into meditation. The bliss must have shown on my face, because the others then sat quietly as well. It was a simple tune, but I was a goner.

Afterwards they set out plates for the meal, began to serve rice and *subji*, but I found it difficult to extract myself from the sweetness of the meditation. I knew I should rouse myself, join them at the table, and I didn't want to be rude; it's simply that the ideation of the song had seized me, taken me into another realm. And I figured that as fellow devotees, they would understand and would cut me slack for a few beautiful minutes more.

For I was already full.

CHAPTER FIFTEEN

It was, in some ways, a simple life in Tiljala: visiting the open-air market—a thriving chaotic organism—to purchase fresh mangos or rice and lentils, taking the breeze on the roof in the evening, figuring out a few chords on the guitar in our room, chatting with passersby. There was a warmth here I hadn't often felt in my own country. A college student walked me through Gol Park one day and wanted to know all about my home village here. Oases of flowers, trees, and ponds placed in the midst of the dust and noise stood out in stark beauty, just as the warmth of the people shone despite the poverty.

On top of this, there were all shades of nationality and personality camped in the jagrti, keeping things interesting. Gregarious Danes, Tamil-speaking grandmothers, Japanese artists, American activists, questioning souls from across every ocean were pulled, perhaps like the young idealists who rushed to fight Franco's fascism during the Spanish civil war; all come to be inspired and work for a set of ideals.

Each morning the heady aromas of cumin and coriander seeped along the corridors of the ashram. Melodies floated from behind closed doors. I woke early, bathed, and climbed to the roof to do an hour of sadhana. After meditation, asanas yoga, it was down to stand in line at the little store carved into the front of the building. Here, next to the small charitable dispensary where villagers received cheap or free medicines, I bought bananas, biscuits and yogurt. Over breakfast those of us staying in the room together got to know each other. "Where are you from? What is AM work like there?"

A monk, already busy with the day's work, might bluster into the room, and apologize for interrupting us. Offered some food, he would reply with that exquisite Indian gesture—hands raised as if in surrender, palms turned outward, head cocked to the side at precise communicative angle, as if to say, "I'm very fine, satisfied, thank you. Please do not inconvenience yourself on my account."

One dada spent the breakfast hour meticulously ironing his uniform. "Baba complimented me," he said, "told me I was the most neatly-dressed acharya." He beamed.

After breakfast it was off to Lake Gardens. Our teacher was a big proponent of physical exercise and went for walks twice a day, morning and afternoon. But if he was busy, which was always, the time for his walk got pushed back further and further, until his morning walk often didn't happen until 1 p.m., and often the afternoon walk was moved to late in the evening. Yet it was during or just after these walks that we might have the chance to be with him and sing together.

In the afternoons, back at the jagrti, I sometimes spent time in the publications department, helping proofread manuscripts. Around five, if it wasn't too hot, I might join in a pickup game of soccer in the open field in front of the building. I sang a few *Prabhat Samgiit* songs before evening sadhana, had a quick meal, and then it was off to see Baba again. Back to Tiljala late into the night, up early the next day, repeat the process.

One day, Baba shook things up a bit by coming to Tiljala. He liked to walk in the garden there, which contained thousands of plants, most of them sent as gifts—ferns with leaves broad as elephant ears, spidery green shoots, sprawling trees, creating a fresh atmosphere and thick as a jungle in places. And flowers: rhododendrons, zinnias, marigolds, lilies, roses. It was one of several botanical gardens Baba had commissioned, with the aim of preserving more biodiversity. Since everything Baba did was both practical and symbolic, I assumed he wanted all margiis to be equally vigilant in protecting flora and fauna.

He walked slowly, leaning lightly on his cane, receiving reports on the condition of all the plants. I watched as he stopped, leaned over and examined one of these plants, cupping it in his hands. He seemed to speak lovingly to a particular flower. Then he called over someone who worked in the garden and asked him a question. The monk responded, and Baba gave instructions about the care of this plant. The dada nodded, jotting some notes in a book. Baba walked on.

The next day there was a tiny new bud on that plant, and when Baba was told of this, he simply said, "I love all things, and I want to see them grow."

Later, I heard that he'd said to the flower, "In this house, you have to follow discipline, little fellow. You have to grow."

One Sunday a friend and I headed to Lake Gardens for Baba's weekly talk. A social worker from Melbourne, Janardhan had red hair, a long beard, and a goofy sense of humor. His rugged good looks, he liked to claim with a grin, "are exceeded only by my humility." Roaming the streets of Calcutta, a space for rumination and friendship opened for us in the midst of the organization's hustle and bustle.

On our way we sprang for a meal at the Maple Leaf Hotel on Park Street. This was a four-star hotel with waiters neatly decked out in shiny uniforms standing discreetly by as the upper-class families of Cal tucked into their large meals. Janardhan and I would spend the equivalent of $8 on a meal there, not a great amount, but a lot for India. Sometimes we just craved a little comfort.

A rickshaw carried us to Ballygunge Market, where we got down beneath a sign hung above one of the shops: "International Sandalwood. Stimulates your senses, Giving You Lasting Happiness and Joy." The famous Bengali sweet shops were here, too, with their abundant trays of sugar-soaked *rasagulla, gulab jaman, jelabi*, a perfect dessert.

Arriving at Baba's house, we parked our slippers amidst the great heap of shoes outside the door, and entered the already packed hall. We found a tiny space, and pulling our knees to our chests, leaned back on those behind us, pressed in like raisins in a box, and still people came squeezing in. But everyone was in a friendly mood, and the ceiling fans swooshed lazily around above.

Janardhan poked me and laughed. "With all the milling around after Baba's talks, sometimes my slippers get snatched up by someone else. I've lost two pair so far. Now I'm trying something new. I place one at one entrance, the other around the other side. Nobody will take just one, right?"

At the front of the room, a heavyset monk, turban slightly askew on his head, pumped the accordion bellows of his harmonium. While waiting for Baba, we sang.

Move along, move along, singing songs. The flame of love is burning bright. All languages, all doctrines, all paths we respect.

A stir. The door on the side of the room opened and Baba entered, walking slowly, resplendent in white. A little ping of recognition rang in my heart. He smiled, a wide, embracing smile. And we perked up. Baba seated himself at the front of the room, and raised his index finger to his cheek. The harmonium dada, taking his cue, began to sing.

Recently Baba had been discussing linguistics. I heard that he'd introduced several new compound letters into the Bengali language, thus addressing some perceived shortcomings of the alphabet. I couldn't conceive of adding new letters to English, but Baba, it seemed, was always thinking outside the box.

Though he often spoke in English, this series of talks was in Bengali, as befit the topic. He began with that mellifluous drawl, and though I couldn't understand what he was saying, it didn't matter. Just watching his face was enough—an eyebrow lifted, a scowl morphing into a grin, then the serenity of his eyes, which reminded me of the telling glance that day outside his gate. His expressions changed quickly; he often seemed to resemble very different persons within a short sequence of time.

A special energy arrived in these Sunday talks. Laying out his theme, Baba told stories, at which the Bengalis rocked with laughter, while we non-Bengali speakers soaked up some of the mood by watching Baba make faces. One story, I learned later, depicted a chance meeting of thieves from different parts of India on a train, who spent their time telling tales of their exploits. The Bengali thief not only had the best stories, but through superior craftiness, managed to cheat the other thieves out of their money.

Perhaps Baba was pricking the Bengali sense of cultural superiority a little with this story. Or perhaps the tale was a metaphor for Baba himself, for wasn't he stealing our hearts? And, he had the best story. "Welcome in the thief," Rumi says, "for he clears your house for the treasures to be had."

Of course, he could be very serious. I heard him speak witheringly about the destructive effects of caste and religious dogma, about the respective failures of capitalism and communism. He regularly instructed people to exercise rationality, to not accept anything blindly. I knew there existed a common misperception of devotees as "blissed-out space cadets," but Baba always emphasized the importance of clear thinking. For someone who might have easily encouraged a personality cult, he did not. This was one of the things that most impressed me about him.

An acharya out for a walk with Baba once pointed out a hole in the road. Baba stepped around it, and then asked, "If I were a sheep and I jumped into a big hole in front of me, what would those sheep following me do?"

"Jump in too, Baba."

Baba was silent for a moment. Then he said, "This is the danger of dogma."

I hadn't yet understood how an immature zeal could sometimes coexist with the expansive benefits of the practice. The possibility that if you were not careful, a sense of self-importance could grow, and arrogance or dogmatism creep in and take root. I would see these pitfalls more clearly with time.

But as my passion for this work was kindled, as I felt my way into it like a young lover feels his way into new depths, I tried my best to see the bigger picture, to understand what this movement was all about. It was what was being shaped, churned, and channeled I wanted to understand. And that seemed to be something broad and deep, a river that flowed within and between us. A river was always changing, always moving. There might be a few backwater pools and eddies, true, yet the river flowed ahead.

On the whole it did its nourishing, irrigating, natural work.

"A sense of call in our time is countercultural," writes theologian Walter Brueggeman. "The ideology of our time is that we can live an uncalled life, one not referred to any purpose beyond our selves." But in this place, at least, a sense of call was the norm.

To monitor the work of the many departments growing under the AM umbrella, Baba had developed a system of taking reports. Each month, at reporting time, the trains into Calcutta were packed with monks and nuns, Baba's workers, streaming in from their places of work from every corner of the country. Each toted their belongings in overnight bags, striding purposefully in resplendent uniforms. And there were the non-Indian acharyas, carefully picking their way, in civilian clothes, through the country's airports.

Ostensibly these meetings allowed the senior workers to review the progress of AM projects. But on another level they were an excuse for people to soak up more inspiration. Baba graced those present with spiritual experiences, answered questions that had often been unvoiced, and rectified mistakes.

He also oversaw the process of posting acharyas to their field of work, a process you could say was a bit different from that of most organizations. Not the most assertive, astute, or even most capable, but often the most devotional person would sometimes be posted in charge of a large project. A young inexperienced acharya might be assigned to head up an entire branch of the organization. Indian Dada, my Bangkok friend, would after a couple of years be put in charge of the mission in East Asia. Baba made the postings based upon criteria most of us could neither see nor understand, the *samskara* or karma of the individual and his or her need for a certain kind of situation in order to grow. Spiritual growth took precedence over anything else. He expected us to learn to swim by leaping into the deep end of the pool.

There were amazing moments. At one reporting session, Baba called forward a young Indian dada, someone whom I'd met.

"You have some pain in your leg, don't you?" Baba asked the young man. This was true; the monk had been feeling discomfort in his knee for some time, though he'd told no one.

"Yes, Baba."

Baba touched the man's knee with his cane. Then he instructed him to leap into the air. According to the stories that circulated afterwards, the dada's knee, whatever its problem may have been, no longer troubled him. This is what I heard, anyway.

It seems funny to say I was developing a deep connection with this man. As of yet, I hadn't even spoken directly with him. I couldn't just go up and say, "Hey, Baba, what's shaking?" Others had a livelier, more conversational relationship with him. Some of the older Indian acharyas, who had been with Baba for twenty or thirty years now, acted freely with him, joking, sometimes even chiding him. I was a minor character, on the margins, not like the senior workers orchestrating this project and that meeting, orbiting faithfully about Baba like so many satellite moons.

But in another sense, in the strange logic of devotion, I felt he was becoming the most important person in the world to me. And I to him. For I could feel that he loved me.

By now I'd heard the highly charged stories of devotees: the woman who dreamed of meeting Baba, seeing his face in a dream, long before even knowing of his existence; the man who saw Baba in a vision, shining with golden light, and merged with him. Such experiences hinted at the deeply mystical and intimate nature of the relationship.

I guess I was embarking on a love affair. The funny thing was, Baba was carrying on such relationships simultaneously with hundreds, perhaps thousands, of others. But I didn't mind. I wasn't jealous. I felt buoyed with energy. My attraction to this man seemed to grow every day through the simplest actions, as I listened to his teachings, read his books, watched him shuffle up and down the path in front of his house. The more I hung out with him, the more I felt a fire being lit underneath my lazy heart.

My Biblical namesake, Andrew, had himself given up a promising career in the fishing industry in order to commit himself to following some strange man he'd had a hunch about. I was on the verge of greater commitment, too. I could feel it. There was, of course, an expectation that the bliss I was feeling would carry a price—that I would be expected to do something in return. That Baba was using himself as a carrot, to get people to work.

I was all right with that. Looking back now I think this is what he meant to impart: *It is for the young to take on the world, to go head to head with it, try to turn it in its rusting axis a little. It took energy and perhaps a little naiveté to think you could change things, and not be too surprised when you actually did, or too downcast when it didn't work out as you'd hoped. The energy of committed young people illuminated the dreams of the world, powering it up like the electric grid of a vast city at night.*

The idea of throwing myself into some work, of maximizing my potential, which seemed obscured beneath the flutter and wow of my insecurities, held a great appeal. I knew there was much I could do in this world, given the chance.

Happiness, I thought, would be to really fulfill my potential.

One day I attended a PROUT rally in a park off Chowringhee Street. Several hundred people milled in front of a stage while a series of speakers thundered their demands into screeching microphones. I kept a low profile on the outskirts of the crowd where one Indian brother tried to translate the various speakers' main points into my ear over the booming of the PA system and the roar of the crowd.

"They are not wanting to allow the wealth generated in Bengal to leak to other parts of India," he shouted. "Bengalis face the problem of economic imperialism—wealth siphoned off to other places by so-called investors."

I'd read something about this. Though having gained political independence in 1948, India was lacking in economic justice. One set of masters—the British—had been exchanged for another—Indian capitalists. Post-colonial history the world over had left the same messy inequities. Countries were mired in a vicious cycle of exporting their own raw materials, then importing the finished products that had been made with those resources. The logic of capitalism compelled it, as corporations sought cheaper labor and fewer regulations wherever they could find it.

The speaker was winding the crowd up now, and my translator tried to keep me in the loop: "We want 100% local employment! Industries should be developed according to the availability of local raw materials! We should not import any finished product that could be locally produced! Protect our local culture!"

Since the mid-1960s, Proutists around the globe had worked to introduce such ideas and to build communities based on these principles. They'd reached out to intellectuals, laborers, farmers and students, envisioning a network of self-sufficient, decentralized economic zones, with local planning, an emphasis on cooperative industry, and ever-increasing improvement in the minimum standards of living.

To move in that direction, Sarkar encouraged the development of high-caliber, ethical leadership and one way to achieve this was through spiritual practice. In this, PROUT struck me as being similar to liberation theology, especially in its emphasis on redressing poverty here and now, not in some vague afterlife.

My own country claimed to have developed an unassailable economic-political system. But it was one that rewarded competition, not cooperation, greed and not generosity. The gap in income levels in the U. S. could only be described as obscene. According to its logic, other nations must either join the ranks of democracy and free enterprise (as if there were a necessary link between the two) or remain undeveloped.

But Sarkar, as early as the mid-1950's, had asked: Why not fully use the resources of a place to create full employment? Why not allow local communities to control their own wealth? Why not resist the notion that the market determines the value of everything and everyone? Why not create a ceiling, in addition to a floor, for the accumulation of wealth? And why not enshrine in each nation's constitution basic economic rights in addition to political ones?

Just as the spiritual philosophy had lit a fire in my mind some months before, I found myself becoming excited about these socioeconomic ideas. I wanted to learn more. And I wanted, maybe, to do some work with the PROUT movement. How that might unfold I didn't yet know.

After the rally, I slipped away from the crowd. Jayanta, the Australian who was writing a book about PROUT, was intent on visiting the offices of *Notun Prithivi*, Calcutta's Proutist newspaper. He invited me along on the half-hour taxi ride. The newspaper was produced the old-fashioned way, the typesetter manually sifting through trays of shiny metal type, lining up the letters, words, sentences and paragraphs of revolution one bit at a time. Writers and editors at the paper took their task seriously, he said, and had made sacrifices. This became apparent when we arrived.

The building was undergoing renovation even as the workers scurried to put out the next day's edition because only a few weeks before it had been firebombed by Communist Party goons. Scorched walls and blocks of plaster flung into corners were physical reminders of the opposition these ideas were stirring. Seeing this, I shuddered. Yet the PROUT workers around me seemed not overly concerned with what had happened. Perhaps they had dealt with it in their own ways, and moved on. After all, they had their work cut out for them. As did I.

CHAPTER SIXTEEN

Floodwaters lapped at the edge of the road, reflections of scattered clouds rippling along their surface. The monsoon rains had been heavy this year and the low parts of the world lay submerged beneath a few feet of water.

Our rickshaw wallah's muscles strained as he pumped his cycle along the elevated highway near Tiljala. Jayanta and I were returning in this cycle rickshaw from Lake Gardens. As we crossed VIP Highway, our driver grinned over his shoulder at us and turned the bike toward the path that led to the jagrti. All of a sudden, losing control, he veered to the right and plunged onto the submerged connecting road. The rickshaw jerked to a halt, and we tumbled into the waters over our heads.

For a brief moment, everything was quiet. Shimmering dapples of sunlight filtered down through murky storm water. Then we emerged from the pool, spluttering. I looked at my friend whose hair lay slicked back on his forehead. He gazed back at me, wonderingly. As the absurdity of the situation—two Westerners and a submerged rickshaw floating in a ditch in one of the poorest wards of Calcutta—washed over us and we burst out laughing. Puzzled by our reaction, the driver hesitantly began to laugh too. Splashing our way out of the ditch, we helped him drag his bike from the mud.

A few minutes later as I dried myself in the sun on our building's roof, I looked out over the sprawl of Calcutta, at the chaotic jigsaw puzzle of houses and hovels hard up against each other; water tanks on roofs, laundry flapping in the breeze. From this angle everything appeared dingy—mottled concrete porches and roofs whipped by decades of wind and rain. The overpasses were dirty white, and everything faded as in an old photograph. None of the buildings looked as if they had been constructed any later than World War II.

A year or so earlier, I'd heard, this little village surrounding our ashram in Tiljala had been badly hit by even bigger floods. Five feet of water had washed over and engulfed the small houses. Many of the villagers sought refuge in the jagrti, and as many as could fit were squeezed into its upper floors. Others camped out on the raised highway and watched their belongings float away. Kindling a bonfire on the road, the dadas and didis churned out thousands of servings of *chapatis* and vegetables over the course of a week. Hundreds of haggard refugees stood in line to receive the foodstuffs in the folds of their shirts. Days passed before the Calcutta government got around to offering any assistance.

The rickshaw incident fit into the nature of things here, just as the flood had: unpredictable, unregulated, tending toward chaos. *How were you supposed to live in such a place?* Juxtaposed with the extraordinary experiences I'd been having with Baba, I felt even more strongly that I was moving through a different world, as if I'd tumbled into a pool, its shimmering waters both sustaining and dangerous. It reminded me of swimming in the ocean, the way the tide pulls your body around and out to sea, swinging you like a needle on a compass.

This concept of fluidity permeated the spiritual culture of India. A word in Sanskrit for devotional love, *rasa*, the flow of attraction, was closely tied to this. It was an attraction you could see in nature, rivers running in high tide toward the ocean, tree sap bearing nutrients to leaves, a child nursing from the breast of its mother. A folk saying about the great teacher Caetanya Mahaprabhu appearing in this region of the world reflected this sense: "Bengal was inundated by a flood of devotion, Santipur was almost sunk, and all of Nadia was swept away by the tide."

I pondered the little village butting up against the highway, the sprawling slums beyond it. Clouds bathed with light shone above the gray aura of the city.

Across the roof from me sat a woman, finishing her sadhana, her legs folded beneath her, hands cupped in front of her chest. She seemed to be offering with an opening motion whatever she imagined was cupped in her hands. Opening, sweeping down, three times she repeated this. Then she sat up, a dreamy, peaceful look on her face. I knew what this was. She was doing *guru puja*, the ritual that completed our meditation, part of the effort to live with an attitude of surrender. If some burden was weighing you down, the problems of the world disturbing your concentration, you could offer it up, release it, visualize it as an offering of flowers, and let it go.

Set it afloat in the river of *rasa*.

One day after the rickshaw incident, I hopped a bus downtown. Diesel fumes wafted through the barred windows of the bus, and passengers squeezed together, hanging tightly to the handgrips so as not to set off a domino effect of bodies tumbling. They seemed to know how to turn within, distancing themselves with ascetic disinterest from their countrymen pressed against their torsos. We passed the square where, a hundred years earlier, the devotional poet Ram Prasad had recited his work before a large crowd, then died. About which it was said, "It was not death. It was translation."

I got down in teeming Chowringhee. A man with eyebrows like bolts of lightning was squatting next to a leaky public tap shaving, peering into a half-broken mirror propped against a building. A cacophony of faces—Mongolian cheekbones, Dravidian foreheads—swept by me. Bolts of cloth jutted from stalls. Riots of figs, dates, cashews, and neat pyramids of oranges, papayas and mangos rose on carts.

A small teashop stood off the street, a wooden shed with rough-hewn planks for tables, beneath a signboard proclaiming "Lal's Restaurant." A counter jutted into the center of the shack, beyond which I could see the kitchen, really just an open fire pit with pots dangling over it. Though I was usually careful about where I ate, I was hungry. I ordered *puris* and *channa*, and sweet yogurt for dessert, and plunked my rupees down. After eating, I nodded to the proprietor and ducked out into the street.

The bookstalls on Free School Street beckoned with their row after row of paperback spy novels—Grisham and LeCarre; dry, imageless tomes on Marxist history; back issues of *Parade* and *India Today*; and comics, *Tintin* and *Asterix*. Students and old men browsed the tables. *Did they wonder about me, about what I was doing in their city?*

Since leaving the restaurant, an uneasy feeling had been growing in me; my digestive fluids were making some rude noises. I sensed the floodgates might be about to open, so I entered a shop and asked for a public bathroom. No luck. I turned and ran into another shop, but again was turned away. Wasn't there a restroom in this whole place? Finally, in one shop a man cocked his arm backwards and pointed. I turned into a narrow dark alley and ran, my stomach in knots. After passing through a series of abandoned rooms—where was the damned thing?—I found it, a smelly hole in the ground.

But it was too late. Before I could reach the toilet, the dam burst. I leaned against the wall, mortified. Calcutta had seized control of my most basic bodily function. Entering the labyrinthine slums of Cal, I had become like a child again.

I cleaned up as best I could, stuffing my underwear into a plastic bag. Then I made my way out of the maze, and, disconcerted, found a bus back to Tiljala.

Along the way we passed the sprawling garbage fill where gulls wheeled, skrawking over a good find. The stench was nauseating. A little further on was the Chinese tannery with its deep and shocking smell of blood and animal flesh. I turned away from the window, pulling my shirt over my nose. The world was conspiring to get under my skin.

Getting off on VIP Road, I ran down the muddy lane to the jagrti, stooping to enter the door in the gate. And just as I made my way across the littered courtyard, the lights in the building went out. I knew this was due to daily slashing of power to spare the city's overworked electrical system but at the moment it was all too much. I ran upstairs, stumbling in the semi-dark, locked myself in a bathroom and leaned against the wall.

God! What am I doing here? Why did everything break down all the time? Why are these people so damned poor?

I picked up a brick of washing soap, frustrated, and began to scrub away at my underwear. Since coming to Asia I'd washed my clothes by hand, had come to enjoy the physicality of it, applying my energies directly to removing the stains and dirt from jeans or shirt or socks, watching the water streaming away change color. The process had a calming effect on me. I began to relax a little. The late afternoon light filtering through the transom, I noticed, was beautiful. It would be time for sadhana soon.

What a struggle to be in this place. Well, all right. Struggle was essential to life. Difficulties and obstacles, Baba had written, were "not to be feared or avoided; rather they are our greatest friends on the spiritual path." This was the tantric way. I was still in enough of a funk to resist this idea. But on some level I felt it to be true. And besides, millions of people lived in conditions like this, I realized, surviving day-to-day, malnourished, their health ruined by pollution, without any choice. *Couldn't I at least adjust my expectations, live a little more in sympathy with the poor? Perhaps work to alleviate some of this suffering?*

How I reacted to the unexpected and the chaotic—to finding myself swimming in a muddy storm-water ditch, or losing control in a crumbling Calcutta back alley—how I dealt with these things was something I had a choice about. Jayanta and I had laughed off the rickshaw incident, and that had felt good. Wasn't it possible to relax into these situations with a sense of humor and empathy for others' suffering?

Maybe.

And Baba was here. Surely there was a reason for that. His words echoed in my ears: "Keep the goal in mind, and move forward." Maybe surrender meant being ready to accept hardship of any kind in the service of a greater goal.

Back in my room, I cupped my hands together, acknowledged the trials of the day, envisioned all of the clashes and aches and frustrations as flower petals lying in my palms. And then I let them go, watched them slide into the surging floodwaters surrounding me.

Chapter Seventeen

David White, in *The Alchemical Body*, writes that the Tantric universe is divine and life-affirming, a pulsating vibratory place in which "matter, souls, and sound are the stuff of the outpouring of godhead into manifestation." It is an emancipating universe. Baba's philosophy affirmed these ideas. But to me, the most important thing was that the philosophy was heuristic, a framework allowing you to experiment with spiritual concepts. Ultimately, practice and experience, not theory, made all the difference.

So I practiced. I sang and danced in the morning, danced and sang in the evening. I sat, trying to corral my restless thoughts and coax my mind deeper. I studied, especially the cogent series of verses expressing the essence of Anandamurti's philosophy in his book *Ananda Sutram*. And I learned more asanas.

I decided to learn all of the forty-some asanas comprising the basic form of AM practice. There were, of course, thousands of asanas developed over the centuries in various traditions. But these forty offered a useful grounding in practice.

I had consulted with several acharyas and been given the go-ahead to learn all of the positions. Now I placed on the floor a book describing the proper method of doing yoga. Printed in India, the book's spine was already nicely broken, and so the pages lay flat. Asana poses were meant to be held comfortably, without straining, but some were easier than others. The *utkata kurmakasana*, difficult tortoise (even it's name suggested difficulty), posed a challenge for me from the beginning. I stretched my body as much as I could, touching nose to toes, cradling my knees in my arms, pressing soles together and thighs to the floor. Pulling one leg up and toward my shoulder, then the other, I was careful not to strain any muscles.

Each day, over the course of my time in Calcutta, those legs inched closer toward their goal—wrapping themselves behind my head. One fine morning both legs slipped into place, I raised my hands together in the namaskar gesture in front of my chest, and my body was a (difficult) tortoise.

Slow but steady wins the race, as the fable goes. Fittingly I seemed to be emerging these days from my shell of shyness, poking my head more and more into the sunlight, my anxieties beginning to dissipate. As I stepped further into this "emancipating universe," a veil seemed to be lifting. A kind of purpose and peace was growing in me, a stability I hadn't known before. It was a great blessing.

West of Calcutta on the desert border with Bihar, sprawled a complex of renewable energy projects, schools, cottage industries, clinics, and spiritual retreat facilities. In this place Tantra was put into practice on a large scale. The growth of *Ananda Nagar*, or City of Bliss, exploded in the mid-80's. I'd heard a lot about the place, and an upcoming Dharma Maha Cakra made for a good opportunity to visit.

It was with a deepening sense of weakness, though, that I arrived at Howrah station. My stomach was still giving me problems, probably because of the Calcutta water. We boiled it, but that didn't seem to help; the stuff was toxic. Though I experienced an occasional sharp jab in my gut, I didn't want to miss this trip, and I made it in time to join other travelers at the station. It had been decided that the non-Indian margiis would travel with a phalanx of Indian acharyas by train several days before the DMC program was set to begin.

As we prepared to leave, the non-Indians were warned again about how Indian police and immigration officials would deport foreign margiis if they caught them. We had applied for and received visas at Indian embassies abroad, and the government had no legal basis to deport us. But at airports and railway stations—those subcutaneous nerve endings of the nation—another, more visceral, logic operated. The government's animosity toward Baba and his progressive ideas had continued into the 80's. Our organization fought the deportation cases in Indian courts and won, but government bureaucrats continued to send margiis packing with a wink between concerned departments. This cat and mouse play added an aura of intrigue to our travels.

So I kept a low profile at the station, nervous but excited. Entering the train and finding our reserved compartment, I bumped into a young man who had his limbs stretched out to make contact with all four bunks. "These are taken," he said. "You want them, you'll have to pay." I was in no mood to argue and forked over ten rupees.

Soon one of the Indian monks entered the car, a mountain of a man. The youth attempted the same scam, but this dada only scoffed at him.

"Dilip! Dilip!" the boy shouted, calling to a crony in another car.

"I'll give you Dilip," Dada said, and closed his hand around the youth's neck. "Don't exploit these good people."

"Dilip!" the boy squawked once more, then bolted from the compartment.

"We are peaceful people," the monk explained to the other passengers who were looking on curiously, "but we won't stand for exploitation." He spread a blanket on the bench and with dignity took his seat.

I fell asleep on my bunk, feverish.

The place I was on my way to visit had not come into being easily. In 1967, five acharyas working at Ananda Nagar had been killed by area villagers plied with alcohol and stirred to trouble by CPI-M, or Communist Party of India (Marxist), cadres. The antagonism of Bengal's Communists toward AM had a long and bloody history. During the national emergency, this same place had been reduced to rubble, destroyed by Communists while most acharyas were in jail or underground.

It would not be the last time margiis were attacked. In Calcutta in 1982, seventeen AM monks and nuns traveling by taxi on their way to Tiljala had been stopped by crowds in what apparently was a coordinated plan, again instigated by CPI-M goons. Acid was thrown into the acharyas' faces. They were beaten with crowbars, their bodies set on fire and they were left to die. The police, bought off, sat on their hands in the station less than a mile away.

This massacre shattered the national news scene. Rallies of condemnation sprang up across Calcutta, and included such public figures as the film director Satyajit Ray. But the West Bengal government dragged its feet; a commission of inquiry was set up, but their conclusions were not released to the public, and no prosecutions were ever pursued. The perpetrators, though never arrested, were known to be local Marxist thugs. And according to several government officials who later came forward, the attack had been part of a planned CPI-M effort to deal with opposition, just as the attacks on Ananda Nagar had been. The orders came from the very top. It was a message to anyone critical of the government: oppose us and this is what will happen to you. Like the pillage of Tibet by the Chinese, *dharma* seemed on many sides assaulted, more often than not by Communists.

However, these days Ananda Nagar was thriving, and AM, its collective sense of Tantric dtermination undiminished, was stronger than ever. Such efforts at suppression seemed only to have backfired.

Jolted awake by the train's slowing, I peered out the window. We were passing through ancient hills marked by the clash of tectonic plates, as if we were moving between geological eras of the earth. Reddish soil shone dully in the moonlight.

The engineer had agreed to stop the train on the other side of Pundag Station and let us jump off so that we could avoid any police dragnet. At the signal, a few groups of six or seven clambered down from the car, clutching their bags, and scrambling across the unknown wilderness. The landscape was pocked with moon craters.

Stumbling through the dark, one brother fell into a small ravine. We heard his cries coming from the earth. Several people rushed to his aid, and, supporting him on either side, they hobbled on. We crossed the sea of sand and upon reaching the outskirts of Ananda Nagar, we were guided to a low-slung building called the Youth Hostel. Exhausted, I threw my backpack into the corner, unrolled a bedroll, and collapsed into deep sleep.

In the morning soprano peals of laughter woke me. I was still a little weak, but overall I felt better. I went outside to take a look around. A rocky horizon stretched before me, marked by the occasional afro-topped tree, terraced paddy fields, shoots of green, and the slip of a crimson sun peeping through the early haze.

Children of the AM school next door were reciting their lessons, twelve kids ranging in age from six to fifteen. I poked my head through the classroom door. A cry went up, but I didn't want to disturb their studies and so withdrew. A little later, at recess time, I came back to take a few photos. Mugging for the camera, the kids tumbled over each other, jockeying to be in front.

They were good kids. The teacher, a young man in his 20's, so short that he barely reached above the children's heads, clearly cared for his wards. He was doing his best to implement the AM educational philosophy: focusing on the needs of the whole child, a curriculum grounded in stories and play, and an early connection to the natural world. It was the basis for hundreds of AM schools around the world. The lessons included English, and several of the children tried out a few words. "Hello, sir. How you?"

I snapped a few more photos with my Dad's old single lens reflex. Its bulky brown leather case was fraying, but it was the same camera he had carried to Brazil, probably the camera with which he'd taken the first photos of me as a baby. I'd seen pictures from that time, snapshots of another poor and rural setting—my brother Bill and sister Susan climbing an abandoned six-foot anthill, Dad standing in front of the jeep that ferried him around the Mato Grosso.

I was, I realized, documenting my adventure in the same way my father had documented his. If I thought more deeply about it, there were other parallels between my parents' journey abroad and mine. They had given themselves to an ideal, and I was on the verge of doing so, too. Of course, the form was not the same, but was the essence so different? Would they, I wondered, have seen it in that light?

Over breakfast, the acharya-principal of the school near where we were staying, his beard covering his face like a forest on a craggy mountain, pointed out some of the highlights of our surroundings: "Eight day schools and night schools for the surrounding villagers, a 40-bed free hospital which is seeing a hundred patients a day, and does free eye operations."

Women in the region, he said, were especially at a disadvantage. The clinics monitored malnourished children and offered free food and vitamins. Instruction was given in gardening, literacy classes, and training of female rural health workers.

As for agriculture, they were working to increase local production through systematic crop planning, harvesting four rice crops a year instead of one or two. This was done through maximum utilization of land and water, and scientific plant breeding.

"This is blowing my mind, Dada," one Italian visitor said. "It's an amazing place."

"Yes, as you say. And it is also a special place in a spiritual sense."

"The hills of Ananda Nagar," Dada continued, "are charged. There were 70 *tantra piithas* here, spots where over the past thousand years yogis had sat for extended periods beneath the shade trees, concentrating their minds." The land itself, he explained, was thus imprinted with a vibrational memory of their efforts. "To meditate on such a spot was a powerful experience; one's mind became instantly concentrated."

I made a note to try this.

For now, though, I wanted to see the river. I walked down the hill, passing Indian devotees clutching shawls and tattered suitcases. Some seemed bewildered by the organization's growth. *Who are all these foreigners? Why is Baba too busy to see us now?* An old woman caterwauled out-of-tune kiirtans, lost in her ideation. The smoke from woodfires drifted across the campus.

I'd heard about the gardens here, blossoming and brambling where before there'd been only dust. Now I looked out over plots of roses, and orchards, too, a litany of green: passion fruit, lichi, papaya, grape, and date palm. Cashew, almond, chestnut, walnut, banana. The area had seen the effects of drought reversed through an intensive water management scheme—proper use of surface rainwater, with small dams creating reservoirs on the rivers, lakes and ponds. As I wandered the grounds, the beauty of the place seemed to coalesce into a harmonious totality. It had not been easy to get here, and the obstacles we'd faced along the way still rankled. But being here was worth it. And tonight there would be another DMC.

I reached the river and waded in, feeling my way along the gravel riverbed. The bed deepened, and so I plunged my head into the cool water. Then I popped up and climbed onto the bank. I was feeling good here in the fresh air and flowing water, as if I'd left the ailments plaguing me back in the city. A flat rock jutted over the bank and I sat down, shivering in the crisp air, water dripping from my body. Up and down the riverbank, people sat on similar outcroppings, deep in meditation.

Several acharyas had washed their clothes in the river, and the brilliant saffron spread to dry, like flame trees dotting the shore, shimmered in the morning sun.

Chapter Eighteen

The heart has its reasons, which
reason does not understand
                              —Blaise Pascal

One Sunday morning a monk poked his head through the door of our room in Tiljala. Seeing us lying there lazily, he did a double take, then shouted, "What are you doing? Baba's calling! Get going—there's a taxi waiting!" Scattering the remains of breakfast and knocking into each other, we managed to gather a few things and run out the door and down to the compound.

The three of us—a young man from New Zealand, another from Berkeley, California, and I—were on the waiting list for Personal Contact. PC was one-on-one face time with Baba. It was said to be a life-changing moment in a margii's life. Baba might offer guidance, he might, through his subtle power, accelerate the exhaustion of your *samskaras*. He would certainly bless you.

If others' experiences were any indication, it was an extraordinary thing. One friend told me about his PC. "I went into Baba's room and Baba told me, 'I want to see you laugh more.' And then he and I just began laughing and laughing, looking into each other's eyes, laughing until the tears streamed down my face. It was beautiful."

It did sound beautiful. I applied, and was put on the waiting list. Each day the three of us made the journey to Lake Gardens, brimming with expectation, where we sat in the hall and read or did sadhana. I used the time to sing more Prabhat Samgiit:

Tumi áshár álo dekhiye jáo ásár kathá bhule' tháka;
You tantalize me with a ray of hope, while your coming remains
uncertain. You keep me holding on. Why do you keep yourself hidden?*

We waited. And waited. Baba was, of course, very busy, but on reflection it seemed our holding pattern itself might have some meaning. Indian devotional literature highlights the longing which Krsna's lover, Radha, experienced while Krsna was away, and she waited for his return. Radha pined and hoped, absence causing her heart to grow exceedingly fonder, until all she could think about and all she saw was his face. Which, of course, was the point—the devotee's consuming need for the beloved elevates his or her mind to new spiritual heights. Baba was stoking our fires.

I was beginning to understand these things. My connection with my teacher was becoming more internal. Not that being with Baba physically wouldn't be extraordinary, but I could appreciate the idea of a gossamer devotional thread, wreathing us together across space and time. Of course, if I *could* have PC, so much the better.

Five days passed, the three of us waiting each day in the main hall at Lake Gardens, seeing Baba on his walks, but not yet entering his room. On this particular Sunday morning we were a little slow getting going. It was unlikely Baba would call for us since he was scheduled to give a public talk later in the day. So we lounged over yogurt and fruit. Suddenly, that acharya burst into our room, his turban half-tied, and sent us packing.

The cab driver had no idea that this was anything other than an ordinary Sunday morning outing. "Faster!" we urged, dissatisfied for once with a taxi driver's pace, but he was nonchalant in his driving tactics as we trundled toward Ballygunge. Halfway there, he stopped to buy cigarettes.

"Are you crazy?" the New Zealander shouted. "Don't you know where we're going?"

Rolling his eyes at these impatient Westerners, the driver calmly opened his smokes, climbed into the cab and we were off again. It was a half-hour ride to Lake Gardens and there we tumbled out, flung 20 rupees at the driver and rushed into the hall.

"We're here, Dada," I said to the man in charge, half-expecting to be ushered right in to see Baba.

"Fine, fine," he said. "Just have a seat."

And so we waited.

Finally, my name was called. Lit with anticipation, I climbed the flight of stairs, turned the corner, and stood in front of Baba's door. Then I took a deep breath and walked inside. What I saw first was that the room was simple and clean, with a few bookshelves and glass cases containing mementos along one wall. But it was also like entering a tunnel;

any image apart from Baba barely registered on my peripheral vision. At the far end of this tunnel, my teacher, my guru, sat on a chair in a corner of the room. He beckoned, and I moved toward him as if through water.

Baba greeted me, asked my name, where I was from. Mysterious great pupils slightly magnified swam behind the thick lenses of his glasses. After a while, he looked off into the air above my head.

I sat and watched him, his eyes flickering back and forth. I had the strangest impression that he was digesting a page out of the book of my life, that he was somehow examining my past. When he spoke, he chided me.

"You have so much potential," he said. "Why are you wasting it?" A tremendous, tender, sadness lay in those eyes.

A litany of the bad habits I'd cultivated in the years before coming abroad sprang to mind. I felt a sense of my own inadequacy, but from Baba I felt no blame, only gentle correction.

Turning the focus away from my shortcomings to what I interpreted as a way for me to move beyond them, he said, "Do something for suffering humanity." His manner was not conversational; this man was serious. And yet as he looked into my eyes, I felt a great love. In that moment I would have gone out and moved mountains for him.

I don't remember making my way downstairs after leaving the room, but my Berkeley friend said that a light shone in my face, as if Baba had kindled something in me. I went and sat for meditation, aware that something momentous had just occurred.

For much of my life I'd been unclear about my place in the world, always concerned about what others thought of me. I'd tried to fill the gaps in my soul with unmindful pleasures. Baba, I think, was reminding me that these tendencies did not represent who I was, in any ultimate sense. They were like the metal filings that cling to a magnet, and I'd found a way to shake them, to move toward an understanding and appreciation of my real self. Sadhana and service—it was so simple. And I was on that path.

I hung around Baba's house all day, attended his talk, gazing goofily at him, and all the while a spark glowed in my chest. I didn't want to leave his house, didn't want him to end his talk. And, later in the afternoon, when an acharya came to me on the street outside Baba's house, saying he had a message Baba had given about me, I perked up.

"Baba said, 'This boy will do some work.'"

Yes.

Something had been building in me over the last several months. Not only had my relationship with Baba flowered, but I was growing to love this organization as well. I wanted to follow through on the promise I'd made to Baba, and do something concrete. It was time to leave India. Seeing Baba one last time I offered him a garland of flowers, which he graciously received.

That same day I flew to Kuala Lumpur, where I bought a ticket for Copenhagen.

I was interested in learning more about PROUT, and LFT (Local Full Timer) training seemed the logical next step. LFTs worked for the organization full-time but were not acharyas, though many of them went on to become acharyas. In Copenhagen, at the world headquarters for PROUT, I would study the spiritual and social philosophies more deeply, and then go on to work as an LFT somewhere, probably in Europe. I relished the thought of the crisp Danish air, of seeing the great architecture of Western Europe, sinking into my Western heritage.

But the Secretary General for the PROUT Department, a towering whirlwind of a personality who happened to be in Kuala Lumpur, had other plans for me. "They're publishing a small PROUT newspaper in Japan," he told me.

"The brother who's been running it is going to acharya training and they need someone to take it over. I'm sending you there."

"But what about my LFT training, Dada?" I asked him.

"*Arre*," he harrumphed, "you'll get your training in the field."

I had slotted myself into the organization, its discipline and its hierarchy, and so I now had to follow its orders. I changed my ticket, as intrigued by the thought of living in Japan as I had been about Denmark, and quietly glad that I was needed somewhere.

PART THREE — TOKYO AND DAVAO

Chapter Nineteen

Brightly tiled roofs under sleeves of snow, patchworks of green fields brooked by earthen walls, small gardens surrounding small shops: a precise landscape, as if everything in it had been thoughtfully cultivated, unfolded before me. In the far distance, I could see snow-capped mountains blooming. And then we were rocketing into the suburbs of the vast city with its kilometers of rabbit-hutch high-rises, small noodle shops tucked into the undersides of trestles, and a sea of neon. Other elevated trains passed us as if in a dream.

Most of the other train passengers—businessmen in suits, schoolchildren in uniform, housewives—had their heads buried in books. I looked around at all these readers and feelings of connection swelled in me. *Oh, land of gentle erudition!* It took a little while for me to realize that most of them were leafing through *manga*, the enormously popular, often salacious, comic books sold in every station.

I would spend two years in this surprising, cosmopolitan and complicated country. Japan would challenge me in ways I couldn't yet fathom. But perhaps most importantly, my life proper within the organization was beginning. I was ready to throw myself into some real work. Ready to set myself adrift in the cosmic flow.

Tucked into my shoulder bag was a letter from my father. I pulled it out and read it through once again.

Dear Andy, My heart is full, but the words won't come—though the tears sometimes do—as I sit here remembering the years of your growing up. All of this to say in feeble words how much you mean to me—to us, as all our children do. I wish I could have been a better father, and example for you.

Nevertheless, we have always desired the best for you, even though our desire and our interpretation of the "best" may not always have been the same as yours! But maybe the "best" includes your freedom, individuality, and independence coupled with the ability, wisdom, and determination to make the right choices and decisions, even though they may be difficult.

He went on to write that he had some concerns about what my commitment to AM might mean to my relationship to the church, and to Jesus.

You should remember your name(s). Names we gave you as a baby in hopes that your namesakes would have an influence on you also. Calvin [my middle name] was a proponent of the sovereignty of God, and one of the founders of Presbyterianism. And Andrew was one of the heart-warming disciples of Jesus.

I don't want this to sound like a sermon or a lecture, but I wanted to express my feelings and remind you of your Roots, and hoped that you would use your head as well as your heart in coming to grips with your future.

He closed by sending his love, hoped that I was avoiding the traveling illnesses, and asked me to write more often. I folded the letter and put it back in the envelope. It was heartfelt. I appreciated that. But it also demonstrated how little he knew me. I was not now leaving the church; I had done that long ago. The fact that he didn't recognize the viability of any other spiritual path bothered me. I didn't feel I was rejecting Jesus; I still respected his teachings. But I had another teacher now. Of course, if my father didn't understand me, part of the blame lay on my side. I hadn't reached out to him, either.

I was distracted, though, from further musing along these lines by the scenes rushing by outside my window. The sparkling impressions of a new world leapt into view around me as our train neared Tokyo Station.

The PROUT office was on the fourth floor of a four-story building in the heart of Tokyo. It was there that I worked with, and grew close to, several men.

Dada BV was an American who sported a long drooping moustache, and when not in acharya uniform, he dressed in black Chinese slippers and soft, flowing clothing, like a Taoist sage. The rich counterpoints of Bach's cello suites echoed from his cassette player. An accomplished artist and photographer, he was related to some famous American writer, although he kept quiet about this. I came to admire him enormously.

There was the Malaysian Chinese monk who possessed lots of devotion but not so much drive. Rolling into Tokyo from tours of other parts of Japan, he often fried up a wok-full of comfort food noodles in the wee hours of the night.

And a young dada from Ghana, friendly and hardworking. He faced a tough time in Japan, where many people had never encountered a black man before. When on occasion he made the rounds of apartment buildings pursuing the tradition of *takahatsu*, or requesting alms, his ebony skin offsetting his striking orange gown, some people slammed the door in his face. He appeared to take it in stride, but I could tell his feelings were hurt.

One other fellow and I became friends, an Indian acharya called IK. As he regaled me with stories of his days in India with Baba, often while whipping up dishes of fried eggplant, bitter melon, and *kichri* in the office kitchen, I found my heart opening, my consciousness sharpening.

We spoke a global glossolalia there, BV and I slipping into ironic American slang: *Yeah, baby!*; the Ghanaian Dada's beautifully eccentric English: *Ohhhh, Yeessss!*;—clipped Cantonese-influenced speech—*Yes lah!*, of the Malaysian, our words flowing into and stumbling over one another as we bent our pronunciations to be understood. Then we would throw in a few stock Japanese phrases, imitating the mock heartiness of sushi shop employees greeting their customers— *"Domo!" "Irashaimasse!"*

These men brought home gifts for me—warm Korean socks, watermelon slices, rice cakes. They took time to talk with me about my spiritual growth, spent evenings with me singing Prabhat Samgiit, suggested readings to supplement my on-the-fly LFT training. All in all, they extended to me the warm love of elder brothers. It was wonderful.

Tokyo, too, was wonderful, and new, and strange. Wandering around our neighborhood I passed restaurants with sliding wooden doors, intricately carved displays of plastic blowfish and *sashimi* in glass cases out front, and flattened myself against alley walls as delivery boys sped by on mopeds, lacquer wooden boxes full of food swinging on scales behind their bikes.

In the small shops, I discovered cardboard boxes with colorful splashes of *kanji*, Chinese characters, brimming with bundles of dark green spinach next to rows of foot-long white radishes. Plastic trays of firm gray tofu still hot from the press and waiting to be carved into blocks, lay next to gorgeous strawberries, Fuji-sized apples, sour plums and sweet persimmons, the blessings of cold latitudes.

Downtown, a square foot of cherry blossom-dappled real estate was worth a million dollars. In the park across from the emperor's palace, kids doled kite line into the sky and office workers in short-sleeve shirts and ties smashed badminton birdies across imaginary nets on their lunch breaks. Sometimes, to get away from the crush of people, I'd pass through a *torii* gate into one of the Buddhist temples or Shinto shrines, into a world of quiet splendor. In years to come Tokyo would haunt my dreams, showing up whenever my subconscious needed to conjure the foreign, the industrious, or the traditional.

But mostly I was busy. Busy, happy, dropping into work. The English-language *Prout Tokyo* newspaper was now my baby, though I received editorial guidance from Dada BV and Dada IK. We published a range of environmental, economic and cultural news in this small paper, a parsing of current events through a Proutist lens. At first amateurish and inky, we discovered we could have it printed on a recently acquired press at another AM office, and it soon began to look more professional.

I set my sights on increasing the circulation, staying up late, rising early, focusing my attention on current events. I'd had, it was true, little training in economics or politics. But I read up. I studied books on PROUT and other topics. I discussed things with the acharyas. If I felt over-whelmed, I remembered my guru's maxim (though it was still strange for me to repeat this phrase, *my guru*. I had a guru!) But I warmed to what he'd said: *The most important requirements for changing society are simply love and a desire to serve.*

Proutist movements promoting economic and cultural autonomy were springing up around the world at this time. In Okinawa, for example, where many locals resented what they saw as exploitation of their natural resources by the Japanese central government, one brother whom I knew was spearheading a campaign to save a fragile coral reef, threatened by plans to construct a larger airport. We highlighted this effort in the newspaper.

I liked the fact that PROUT offered both an inspiring vision— one human society moving together toward a common goal—and a practical set of economic ideas. Did I wonder, sometimes whether PROUT would ever be accepted on a larger scale? Of course. One or two Proutists had been elected to office in India, and there were grassroots projects in some places. What we had, mainly, was an understanding that such larger-scale impacts were both needed and possible. Needed because the systems now in place were despoiling the planet and leaving half its population in poverty. And possible, since history demonstrated that whenever regimes became too oppressive, change happened.

I was stepping into that stream of idealism in Tokyo, adding my candlelight to the sum of light. I plugged away, inspired by memories of my recent time in Calcutta, and by the others in the office. At the photocopy shop down the street, jostling with scores of university students copying their textbooks, the smell of toner thick in the air, incomprehensible Japanese announcements tacked to the bulletin board, I enlarged the paper's headlines to their proper size.

Hidai thus became one of my first words of Japanese. To expand.

A lot of money was required to support the clinics, schools, and development projects taking off in India and other places. Margiis gave donations, but these often weren't enough to fully fuel the humming machinery of good works. Acharyas working in wealthy countries like Japan were thus expected to help finance these efforts, in addition to whatever local projects they were overseeing. Facility in making money was, perhaps unexpectedly, a valued skill among the monks and nuns.

One such effort I admired was a benefit concert being organized to raise money for Burkina Faso, the eastern African country where a clinic and anti-desertification program served 17,000. Dada Dharma, an American monk who worked as Public Relations Secretary for AM in East Asia, oversaw much of the preparation for this event. He had enlisted several popular Japanese musicians as performers, and hoped to raise enough money to send a tractor to Africa.

I heard a lot about plans for the concert since on Sundays, after group meditation, I usually slept over at the AM office in Nakano-Fujimicho. We had great breakfasts there—rice crackers draped in dried seaweed and flecked with sesame, salty *misoshiro* soup and glutinous rice cakes. Conversation at breakfast usually included one or two Baba stories, but it also centered on work.

Sometimes there were clashes. One morning the office secretary, an Argentine named Dada Shakti, called Dharma into the office. A clamor could be heard, the two men shouting at each other.

"I need RS to focus on his duties!"

"And I need him to help with the concert!"

"You are always micromanaging!"

Dharma stomped out of the office, grabbed his jacket, and left the jagrti, slamming the door. Shakti came into the room, shaking his head. After a while, he laughed.

"You know," he said, "he's a great man."

There were disagreements in the PROUT office, too. Hunching over a desk reviewing articles for the next edition of *Prout Tokyo*, I eavesdropped one morning on several of the acharyas arguing about tactics. Dada BV had begun to push the envelope of monastic behavior by carrying duty-free whiskey and cigarettes to sell in the black market when he traveled to Korea. He often rode the bullet train without buying a ticket. This, one of the others said, was conduct unbecoming of a monk. "No," BV countered, "it's necessary, since money is so tight."

I was beginning to see that people embraced the revolutionary identity of AM in various ways. One was in accepting a certain level of creativity when it came to raising money. Tantriks, the reasoning went, were willing to take risks, embrace the unorthodox if necessary, provided they kept their spiritual goal fixed before their eyes. But it was possible to get carried away when it came to moneymaking ideas, to be swayed by the enthusiasm we felt for the work.

"The thing is," Dada IK, the Indian monk, told me later, "Some things can tarnish the reputation of the organization. We are doing so much service; our reputation is important."

"Live your life according to spiritual principles," he said. "You'll manage. Baba is with you."

IK had wonderful memories of growing up amidst the resplendence of the North Indian fields. And of becoming a margii at age 13, though his parents were opposed to it. He went to live in the jagrti in Ranchi, during a period of government repression. The police raided the jagrti, and arrested him and others for simply being margiis, and he remained in jail from 1971 to 1973. But, he said, "We had such a high spiritual life at that time, singing and dancing in the prison, that it was easily bearable."

Another of his stories amazed me. He'd been posted to South Korea and, never having been to a cold country, didn't know how to cope with the severe weather. His feet became frostbitten, and for months severe pain affected his legs. Bedridden, he was lonely most of the time, he said, since there were few other acharyas or margiis in Korea then.

One day, while he was resting, he heard the sound of someone cooking. He opened his eyes. Baba was standing at the stove, preparing food.

"You're weak," Baba smiled. "Please don't move."

Stunned, Dada asked, "Baba! When did you come?"

"A little while ago. You were sleeping so I didn't wake you. I've just come from Calcutta. It was a long journey, so I was getting something to eat."

"You were feeling lonely," Baba continued, "so I had to come see you physically. But why feel lonely? Don't you know that I'm always with you?" Dada closed his eyes and sank into an ecstatic state. When he opened them Baba had disappeared. He was happy to have seen him but wept bitterly that he was gone.

What could I say to such a story? Was Dada feverish, only imagining that Baba had come to visit him? Was it a mystical vision? Was it an example of our guru's incredible capacity for love, that when one of his beloved devotees needed him, he came? I don't know. But I do know how the story made me feel.

Six months after I arrived in Tokyo, our office lease expired and the landlord, hoping to raise the rent, forced us to move. We found a new apartment not far from Shinjuku, a major transfer point for rail travel to points west. Once a bohemian center—haunt of students, artists, and radicals—Shinjuku was increasingly being transformed into a gleaming business hub. It was also the site of a homeless hot-meal project we organized.

Many Japanese claimed there were no homeless in Japan. Nevertheless, in the arteries of the great station a cardboard box community had sprung up, inhabited by hundreds of people in grimy clothes, some of them mentally disturbed, claiming their five feet of space for their crusted cardboard homes as commuters strode by, ignoring them. On the whole they were gentle and polite. We carried hot soup, rice, and pickles to a nearby park, and shared these to lines of the forlorn-looking men, following Baba's advice to "give respect to those whom society does not respect." In colder weather, we gathered in the covered areas leading from the streets to the stations and handed out blankets.

I remember one man, seemingly unwashed for days, the smell of urine and alcohol radiating from his mismatched clothes, standing shyly in line, unable to meet my gaze. But when he received his tray, the slightest hint of a smile crossed his face.

All this was eye-opening for me. I'd naively never conceived of the existence of mental illness or grinding poverty in Japan. The experience helped me to see the universal humanity in these men—any human mind in the wrong circumstances was liable to drop into paranoia. Or in the right situation, to find peace. So much depended on context.

We were inspired in this work by Sarkar's latest book, *The Liberation of Intellect: Neo-Humanism*, which critiqued the human tendency to focus on limited circles of concern: family, or city, or region, or nation, or religious grouping, to the exclusion of others. We all read it and discussed Sarkar's emphasis on the importance of nurturing 360-degree vision. The philosophy of neo-humanism was so-called because it went beyond the classical "humanism" espoused in the 17th and 18th centuries, a humanism that shifted emphasis away from God (and the excesses of institutionalized religion) toward human needs. That trend was anti-clerical, but threw the spiritual baby out with the bathwater. This "new humanism" was both spiritually and ecologically attuned. Plants and animals had their existential value, too; they weren't on the planet simply to be used by humans.

The book also pointed out how political leaders played on people's sentiments in order to consolidate power, and offered strategies for counteracting these ploys. When enough people started to break free of limited sentiments, this would create a tremendous wave in the collective mind. And this would naturally lead to social change.

BV organized a series of events to highlight these ideas. At the first evening, fifty people showed up at the public hall we'd rented. With his usual flair, BV had put together a slide show on the state of global economics. When a photo of the G-7 leaders—Reagan, Thatcher, Nakasone—flashed on the screen, a jeer went up from the international crowd. These people liked what we had to say about a more cooperative economics. After dinner, a margii performed an original song, "Take your love and learn to fight." As he sang, a half-Japanese, half-African-American two-year old toddled out in front of the audience, hanging her little head left, then right, in time to the music, bringing gales of affectionate laughter from the crowd.

Back at the PROUT office, we debriefed. The evening was deemed a success. BV turned to me. "You should host the next one."

I swallowed. "What! But I'd be really nervous."

"I was nervous, too," he said. "You can use that nervousness, turn it to your advantage. Like any energy, it can be redirected."

What could I say? I was here to face my fears. I'd always had anxiety about how I was perceived. I never wanted to put myself into a situation where my weaknesses might become known. But BV reminded me that our path was about living out of spirit, not ego. And shyness, too, could be a manifestation of ego, a preoccupation with self.

So a few weeks later I helped set up the hall on the evening of the second event, and then strode out before the crowd of 30 or so and announced the program. Inwardly I was shaking. But Irish Dada played a reel on his fiddle, the LFTs from the other offices whipped up an incredible meal, and people seemed to be enjoying themselves. It was no replication of the first evening's outstanding success. But it wasn't bad. I did all right. And it was a step for me—an important step.

In fact, things were shifting in Tokyo. Increasingly I could see the benefits of meditation etched in my psyche. I was growing in confidence, able to drop my bundle of insecurities sometimes and experience unencumbered joy. Earlier in my life I felt like I'd been living under an eclipse, some dark body casting over my personality a ghostly filtered twilight. Now it had begun to pass, my inner light to shine more freely.

"Hey!" one Japanese sister exclaimed after seeing me sitting quietly for months, and now beginning to interact more with others, to take initiative. "You've changed!"

Autumn arrived, gorgeous crimson leaves on the beech and maple trees dropping to the sidewalks. The little sweet shop across the street offered leaf-shaped candies to commemorate the season. Pat Metheny's bright guitar licks rang out from the cassette deck in our office, alternating with Prabhat Samgiit, both sounding notes of optimism.

During this period I met Ryuku-san, a five-foot tall Zen monk. In a way, he became a mentor, too. With his shaved head, swirling grey robes, sparkling eyes and tiny stature, he was like a creature from another world. Ryuku spoke little English, my Japanese was scanty, but somehow we managed to understand each other. He meditated in a monastery during the winter, but in the off-season he was free to do as he pleased, so he often came to the PROUT office for lunch, intrigued by these Western monks.

One day while he was visiting we heard the rumble of heavy machinery outside the window and ran downstairs together to watch the bulldozers demolish an aging building down the street. Wrapping his fingers through the loops of the chain-link fence, he told me he'd loved playing with Tonka trucks when he was a boy.

"Hey, me too!" I exclaimed.

Ryuku-san was always trying to get across to me the nature of Zen. Waiting until my guard was down, he'd shout, "Now!" as if trying to cure me of hiccups. "This is moment! Nothing else, only this moment!" Laughing at his tactics, but grateful for the reminder, I rolled my eyes. He grinned, and we turned back to watch the towering crane scoop its payload of dirt into the beds of the rumbling dump trucks.

Ryuku reminded me that Zen had laid claim to the Western imagination in a way few other Eastern disciplines had. The Beat poets of America—Jack Kerouac, Allen Ginsberg, Gary Snyder—probably helped more than anyone to spread its ideas in the U. S. I admired the hint of irreverence in Zen, epitomized by the perhaps apocryphal story of the monk who burned a Buddha statue to keep warm during a frigid winter. Zen's aesthetic seemed to appeal to a Western sensibility overwhelmed with information.

Interacting with Ryuku helped me to place my own practice into context. What I understood was that Zen worked on emptying the mind, slicing away defining or constraining idea, and in their place offering pure being. Tantra emphasized filling the mind with awareness of a deeper reality—the fact that all was God—and the heart with love.

Like Zen, Tantra offered as part of its practice the chance to fight against negative mental energies. Also shared was a commitment to the *dharma*—underlying essence and guiding principle—a common heritage. And finally, they both understood that ultimately one must surrender, let go, the hardest thing of all.

Ryuku-san wondered if I was attracted to the life of a monk. Surprisingly, he advised against it. "You will do more as ordinary person. Fit better without monk uniform." I later learned that he was being pressured to serve as head priest of a nearby temple, a prospect he greatly resisted. He wanted to remain footloose.

But his advice did give me pause. It's true that the acharya's uniform elicited reactions. Once the American monk, Dada Dharma, and I were walking in the mountains. A Western hiker came up and, taking in Dada's robes and turban, screeched: "Why do you have to wear that? Fine, teach yoga, but why do you have to wear something so weird?"

This guy seemed uptight about the disjuncture in psychology involved in putting on the saffron robe, in stepping away from the ordinary. Yet such symbolic provocation was also part of its beauty. As Dharma pointed out, the uniform was meant to be eye-catching, to draw attention to the ideals—service to humanity, commitment to a higher vision. Of course, it *was* a little strange for a Westerner to wear these robes, from a certain perspective. But the uniform was the outer layer of a radical commitment. Part of that commitment was letting go of what others might think of you.

Could I see myself wearing the acharya uniform? I didn't know. Yet I was beginning to think more seriously about the possibility.

CHAPTER TWENTY

She was the most beautiful woman I'd ever seen. Or maybe it was just that desire tends to express itself in absolutes. More than beautiful, she was funny and effusive and I loved this. I was often attracted to women who were outgoing, believing they could pull me into their extroverted world.

And I felt this way about Maria, though we barely knew each other. With her long auburn hair and green saucer eyes, the twenty-something Spanish girl studying Montessori education methods here in Tokyo was driving me crazy.

On Sundays we crossed paths in Nakano-Fujimicho at the weekly meditation circle. Casting about for something to say, I asked her about her studies. Maria tucked strands of red hair behind her ears and smiled sweetly at me. "Eet ees going hokay," she said. This simple exchange fortified me, left me wanting more. I looked forward to Sundays when I could sit across from her, perhaps catch the scent of her perfume.

Who knew? Maybe, with time, we'd find we had a lot in common. Maybe I came to Japan because I was supposed to meet her. Maybe...

Thus careened the smitten musings of my mind.

Despite this, I was a Local Full Timer (LFT), and shared some of the conduct rules with acharyas, which included celibacy. This would, of course, preclude pursuing a romantic relationship with the red-haired girl, or with any woman. How could these two facts coexist in one body? Yet with the dazzling incongruity of human life, they simply did.

I had lived in Tokyo for almost a year. Each morning at the PROUT office we rose and sat for an hour in reverent silence as the sun peeked over the Shinjuku skyscrapers surrounding our building. I enjoyed soaking up the dadas' energy. I admired their commitment. I dipped my toes gingerly into this pool, sometimes considering whether I might want to take the next step and become one of these robed figures.

Although many would resist the notion, there were solid arguments in favor of celibacy. It wasn't just discipline or denial for its own sake. Like fasting, such a commitment could allow for a clearer mind, a chance to immerse yourself fully in a creative undertaking (in this case, spiritual practice) without the, shall we say, *distractions,* inherent in a sexual life. Acharyas and LFTs gave themselves fully to the work. Such a commitment brought you to a place where you were able to acknowledge the deeper qualities of those around you, to see people's sacred nature, not just their sexual appeal.

Still, much of the world seemed to react with locker-room incredulity to a person who would not pursue sex, given the chance, who would set those energies aside for other purposes. Even St. Augustine had been ambivalent on this score, praying, "Lord, grant me chastity and self-control. But please, not just yet."

As I grappled with the options, the question arose: how fully can you understand yourself if sexuality, an integral part of human life, is removed from your experience? It's true that a few monks I'd met seemed ill suited for the celibate life. They tended to be dismissive of women in a way that suggested a fair amount of self-repression at work. But, sublimation and repression are not the same thing. Many other acharyas I knew had learned to channel their desire into something else, and seemed quite happy, more than happy, with their life choice.

I'd already had some sexual experience. In college the white noise of sex had hung over the air of the campus like a low electrical hum. I dated a few women during those years, but didn't seem to be built for a longer-term relationship. I remember a woman whom I saw for a few months at Trinity. We were both lonely, it seemed, both wanting love, but she was also flighty, and I insecure. We tumbled into the stage of physical intimacy. It was a good experience as far as it went, but I hadn't yet realized that I was going about things backwards. That love was supposed to precede sex.

I was certainly attracted to the curve of women, to form as beauty. And I searched for perfection within that form, for some answer to my confusion, though, of course, it was not to be found. For how could flesh alone solve a problem of the spirit?

So in Tokyo I knew what I would be putting aside as I contemplated celibacy. And on good days I suspected that the joy of dedication to something greater than my own needy self would more than make up for the loss of intimate connection.

And yet, the mountain that was desire rose ever within me, subtly shifting its slope, ready to unleash a mudslide to level my carefully constructed house of restraint. Sometimes my longing seemed as solid and ever-present as that actual great mountain, Fuji, which thrust itself into the sky on the outskirts of the city.

Tokyo was a glittering field, a city of distractions and temptations. Skyscraper nightlife blared and beckoned. Millions of beautiful women strolled the streets.

Maria showed up every Sunday and smiled at me.

The PROUT office floor was covered with traditional *tatami* rice-straw mats. They were clean and soft, two to three inches thick, creating a space conducive to reflection.

One evening a friend paid a visit. He was an LFT, like me, living at another AM center in town, and also considering becoming an acharya himself. We sat on the *tatami* and ate rice and vegetarian sushi, and he talked about growing up poor in France. Later, the topic of conversation shifted to his feelings for a certain cute Japanese woman we both knew. He was enraptured. Another thing we had in common.

Becoming animated as he described his feelings, he clutched his fork in one hand. Suddenly, he lashed it into the *tatami* mat a few inches from my hand. *Sproing!*

"This is what I feel, the intensity of it!"

The fork trembled in the *tatami*. I stared at him, startled. After a moment, he relaxed and apologized. He'd only been making a point.

"Maybe you've been working a little too hard," I said.

The thing was, you couldn't let things get out of control. We both knew this, that sometimes desire could be overwhelming. Beneath the surface of everyday life, collusion existed between head and heart and organ, a feedback loop wending through poles of environment, memory, desire and physical sensation. Raise any of these factors to a higher level, and a young man's body found itself in a swarm.

After all, these were heavy biological forces at work. The full brunt of the evolutionary impulse was transposed, so that we explicitly did not ignore it, into pure pleasure coursing through the body.

In yoga physiology terms, the problem indicated an imbalanced *svadisthana* or second cakra, one of the psycho-spiritual energy centers, operating within a complex symphony of glands, hormones and external stimuli. It was necessary to bring this cakra back into balance.

For this, there were measures you could take, the yogic version of a cold shower. Food to avoid, exercises to perform, tight-fitting *laungota* underwear to wear. Fasting, said to redirect excess spermatic fluid in the body, helped, as did immersing yourself in work. The dadas' example demonstrated to me that when passions were brought under control, a deeper, less distracted, enjoyment of life was possible. This was no Army-Corps-of-Engineers wholesale damming of desire, but a skillful irrigating redirection of energy to higher faculties.

It struck me that the idea of masculinity, of mastery, that I'd latched on to in Texas—that being a man meant one should be able to attract women by being in control—was turned on its head. Not to be at the mercy of desire, to control oneself through spiritual practice, this was the paradigm now being offered to me.

But there was also a funny paradox—despite our rigorous practices, ultimately we could never really be in control at all. Something would always challenge the assumption of control, some pebble flung by a passing car wheel would plunk into and roil the waters of our serenity. Accepting the need to let go, even of being in control, seemed an important lesson, yet one that I had not yet fully grasped.

I spent a lot of time underground. Tokyo was an expensive place to live, and some acharyas had discovered a creative money-making venture to help pay expenses. They set up small stands in obscure corners of subway stations evenings and sold imported goods—oil paintings from Korea, Indian clothing, arts and crafts. I began to do this, too.

Japanese society in the 1980s was shaped by prosperity, youthful energy, and an unshakable drive for work. As millions commuted to their jobs, doing their part for the national boom, they passed through the huge humming subway stations of the city and its sprawling suburbs, stood waiting on the train platforms, practiced their golf swings with invisible five irons. Sometimes they bought my wares.

After a day working at the PROUT office, I sat quietly in meditation, struggling to withdraw my thoughts from the material plane. Then I ate some dinner and descended into the steamy Tokyo underworld.

As I headed downtown, a gentle electronic female voice cautioned me at the stoplight to wait until the light changed. Another feminine voice invited me to watch my step please while getting on and off the escalator. On my way to Shimbashi station, I passed rows of *pachinko* players sitting amidst a mesmeric haze of cigarette smoke and staring at the steel balls springing around and around in the glass case. Lights flashed, bells rang. Despite the crowds, I sensed a great loneliness there.

As I set up my painting stand, people sauntered over and squinted at my collection: Parisian street scenes with streetlights reflected in puddles of rain, dabs of oil forming blue ocean swirls. Sometimes they struck up conversation in their limited English. Or I trotted out my slowly expanding bag of Japanese phrases.

"*Kombanwa. Homono e desu.*"

"Berry Gooo! Berry Gooo! Where you from?"

During slow times I read a book by Takeo Doi. He wrote that human feeling and social obligation were so intertwined in the Japanese that to be isolated was the same as losing one's self. I watched the faces rush by and knew what it was to be an outsider.

Sometimes I wondered if Maria might happen by, even though I knew that was unlikely in this city of 20 million. What a beauty she was. If only we could spend more time together. How nice it would be to talk with someone who understood what it was like to be young, looking for something, and not from here.

But she was busy, and so was I. And so our acquaintance never seemed to progress beyond exchanging a few words at the meditation meeting. In fact, I hadn't seen her for a few weeks. She probably had no idea how I felt about her.

Toward ten o'clock, the energy of the station shifted. A drunken businessman ran down the stairs and danced in front of my stand, knocking over some of the paintings. In the underground transfer passages, lithe arms and elaborately colored lips from billboards reached out to embrace me. Forty percent of the people who passed were female. Tokyo is a fashion hub, where women pay attention to how they look. Despite myself, I paid attention to how they looked, too.

One of the acharyas had remarked to me that when you see clearly, desire fades away.

When I see clearly? Really, for me at this point in time wasn't it about not seeing at all? Employing the redirected gaze? *Do not look, do not look.* Simple as that, do not look, and cut yourself free from the entangling mesh of desire. Do that and the whole damned dog and pony show never gets a chance to roll into town.

I looked anyway.

Sometimes, the clamor of my sexual desire seemed a clamor against loneliness, against the fear of not being loved. Lust, of course, played a part. But lust, I was learning, could with some effort be redirected into other energies. Loneliness was a spiritual matter.

Life in Tokyo had helped me to grow up a little. My conception of what it meant to be an adult, to be a man, had shifted. I'd begun to ponder some of the deeper questions about my place in the world, about my relationships to others. And yet, desire was still there. When I thought of the Spanish woman, I wanted her.

Families returning from Tokyo Disneyland passed by, their sleepy children clutching helium-filled Mickey Mouse balloons. Of course, I knew there was a distinction to be made between sexual attraction and loving relationship. And a celibate life would also mean cutting myself off from the deep playfulness and affection of being with someone, or of having children. Did I want to give that up?

Snow was falling over Tokyo as I returned home from the subway, drifting in silence through the circles of light cast by streetlamps. At home I sat on the floor and closed my eyes. The *gomukhasana* exercise was supposed to help control sexual desire. Crossing one knee over the other, I stretched my right arm over my shoulder, while my left arm reached up behind my back to grasp it. As my body pressed into it, the *tatami* mat released a sigh.

When Dada BV came into the room the next morning, he cleared his throat, then told me that Maria had left Japan, had flown to England to work in a preschool, moved on in her youthful search for adventure. I felt as if a pair of pliers had reached out and given my heart a twist. What the hell? I'd never had a chance to say goodbye.

My future had not yet swum into focus. I didn't know if I would go on to become an acharya. I didn't yet know if I made the commitment whether I would discover within me the energy necessary to sustain a celibate lifestyle. Would it work for me?

On this wintry morning in Japan, none of that was yet clear, and I was missing Maria. But what could I do? I silently wished her well. Then I turned to look out the window at the vibrant, teeming city, taking a moment to drink in the world before the time for meditation rolled around again. The great mountain in the distance thrust itself through a layer of clouds, very visible today.

Chapter Twenty-One

"Not wholly dark nor shining bright, but softly glimmering. Oh beautiful beyond compare, the misty moon of a night in spring."

Japanese poet Chisato could have been describing the glittering night above Mt. Fuji, which, at 12,388 feet, dominates the horizon of the central Japanese plain. In the indigenous Ainu language, Fuji means "to burst forth." It's a mountain of mythic proportions, the inspiration all Tokyo strains to see. Buddhists in earlier times believed that to set foot on the peak was to acquire good karma, a better rebirth. These days many older people see the climb as a pilgrimage of the Shinto faith and the whole of Fuji is considered a Shinto shrine. Even young Japanese who've eschewed religion wholesale seem to find deep meaning in the experience. For me, some months after Maria left Japan, it was no longer desire that the mountain symbolized, but transcendence.

I'd always loved the high places of the world. If offered a choice between living by the ocean or by the mountains, I knew which one I'd pick. This mountain had been calling to me since I'd arrived in Japan. On a smog-free day, Fuji presented itself like a work of art on Tokyo's western horizon, and I relaxed for a moment and drank in its beauty. Fuji added soul.

So one cool evening, four male friends—an Indian acharya, a visiting Hong Kong margii, a Japanese acquaintance and I—made the journey to Fujinomiya, "place of seeing Fuji," in hopes of having the mountain's *darshan*.

We had decided to make our ascent during the night, mostly because we wanted to experience sunrise in this land of the rising sun from Japan's highest vantage point. Fuji was divided into ten stations and most climbers drove to station number five near the timberline to begin the trek. Our taxi driver dropped us off at the fifth and wished us luck.

I was turning over a question in my mind.

The moon was full, though obscured at times by clouds. At such moments our pocket flashlights were the only means of picking out the trail. Of course, the only way to go was up, and we moved ahead on the lava-strewn path, talking sporadically, enjoying the night's silence. At the sixth station we reached the timberline, where foliage was sheared off the land like the sharpened tip of a pencil. This made it easier to see, but also meant having to deal with a bone-chilling wind whipping down from the rocks above.

Two Japanese college students sat on the path before us puffing on cigarettes after a long climb. Crazy kids.

Konbanwa.

Konbanwa.

They finished their smokes and strode on ahead. Our group took a break, settling on some flat rocks.

The question I was considering was this: should I go to acharya training? I had lived with acharyas in Bangkok, Malaysia, and Calcutta, and now in Tokyo for close to three years. I was attracted to the life. But was I cut out for it? I needed to analyze my motives. Was part of the attraction simply because I had earlier been so adrift? Was I longing for a structure I had never known? No, that was too simple. And besides, I was no longer that person.

I'd read a magazine describing an especially well-liked monk in India: "Acharyaji is honest, disciplined, respected by all. He wakes in the silent atmosphere at 4 a.m. without fail. He strictly performs his spiritual practices at the proper time. He lives a well-routined life, is never idle, and is dedicated to service." Such a life spoke to me. The principles which AM espoused appealed to me, too. It was a wonderful ideology. And I loved the dynamic monks and nuns, the activist margiis I'd met. Didn't it make sense to commit more deeply to this family?

And yet, how would my family of origin react to such a decision?

I could have gone back to the States, gotten married, and tried to integrate what I'd learned into an ordinary life. Most members of AM were family people, not monks and nuns, after all. But the strong sense of fulfillment I felt these days was pushing me toward something more.

And besides, the renunciation I was considering wasn't a negative one, not some self-incarceration in a Himalayan fastness to subsist on a diet of slugs and yak butter. I would later read what Kathleen Norris wrote in *Dakota*: "Asceticism is not necessarily a denigration of the body, but a way of surrendering to reduced circumstances in a manner that enhances the whole person." This, I realize now, squared with what

I was learning. Such a path asked you to serve the world. And if I took this step, I would be living in the thick of that world, wherever I ended up.

And yet. And yet, my ancestors lived in me. Their stream of faces reached back from my father and mother to each of their fathers and mothers and beyond, their wonder, promise, despair, all genetically coursing through my body, shaping the way I spoke and moved and thought. My grandfather, Baptist minister, was in me. I was part Scottish, part English, my ethnic background so much a foreground in my home country that it disappeared into itself. Would I be turning my back on all this?

Since they were posted to foreign lands, many AM acharyas didn't see much of their blood family, sometimes for years. This was rooted in the renunciation tradition of India, of completely giving up the things of the world. Some did try to keep in contact with family members. But there was something about the commitment that seemed to prompt new acharyas especially, in their early years to be more rigorous in their separation.

I knew such a decision would probably cause my parents pain, and I was sorry for it. As I look back now, I see that I left some work undone, that I had never really gotten to know them, adult to adult. We had unfinished business. I would be skipping that phase and the potential resolution of our conflicts.

Yet I'd come abroad, I reminded myself, because I needed a radical change in my life—the gaps in my self-awareness had been too great back in Texas.

If ordinary life seemed a judicious lab exercise that followed the instructions closely, I'd instead been looking for explosions and foaming beakers, groundbreaking discoveries, an elemental alteration of my way of thinking. And this is what I'd gotten.

The wind continued to sweep down the mountain. Around three a.m. an outcropping rose in our path and our group decided to stop and try to get a little rest. Huddling together for warmth, we dropped into an uneasy sleep for an hour or so.

The shifting grayness of dawn nudged me awake. I sat up and woke my friends. Since the top was still some distance away, we decided to enjoy the sunrise from the ninth station, an hour's walk from the summit, just a few minutes from where we'd slept. We sat on rocks and watched the show. Far out over the Pacific, a sketch of intense color was unfolding: shifting purple transforming into orange, then fiery red hues at the indistinct line where steely sea met murky sky.

Soon a bright orb of orange slipped over the horizon, extraordinarily large from this angle. The Indian dada, always sentimental, sang out, "Lord, thank you for this beautiful morning!" I sat for meditation, feeding the natural high with an internal high. And afterwards, as I opened my eyes, enveloped by sun, sea, and sky, things suddenly became clearer. The simple fact of Anandamurti's existence, his example, was the real incentive to become an acharya, and an extraordinary one. If becoming an acharya meant I would have the chance to get closer to Baba, this was a beautiful thing.

By now it was six a.m. The mountainside below had transformed into a mosaic of motion as dozens of early-bird climbers hiked upwards. More than half of them were over the age of 60, radiating robust health. A young man with a lightweight ten-speed bike strapped to his back strutted past us. Cheerful camaraderie emerged. "*Ohayo gozaimasu*," we bid each other good morning, or "*Ganbatte kudasai*"—"Show that indomitable fighting spirit!"

Rubbing shoulders with the other hikers, I felt I had broken through some longstanding cultural barrier. And in an hour we were at the summit, whooping our triumph into the dormant volcanic pit.

Chapter Twenty-Two

The earth circled its star twice while I was in Japan. The Eighties were slipping by. Back in the States, an unsettling political conservatism had settled in. How else to explain the election, and more striking, re-election of Ronald Reagan? In much of the Midwest, the farm crisis was shaking rural life down, throwing multiple generations of farmers off their plots, the land falling under corporate ownership. Reagan was busy setting a deregulatory precedent that would radiate troubling consequences for American society for years to come. He had declared that it was "morning in America," but I feared it was a gloomy twilight.

My family members were all getting on with their lives. My sister, a church musician, was raising a family of three wonderful children with her husband, a Presbyterian minister. My brother had for some time been active with progressive causes, and had even made a run for U. S. Congress on the Socialist Party ticket. He had now started an organization called Criminal Justice Ministries, which advocated for prisoners' rights. My father had found work as a computer technician in Dallas, my mother as a librarian at an osteopathic college in Fort Worth.

I suspected, though, that my parents were worried about my long absence. Why would I go to live overseas without even finishing my college degree? Dad's earlier letter had revealed some of their concerns. To have no career in the conventional sense, how must that have looked?

I got the chance to find out. Another letter arrived from my parents, saying they would be visiting my aunt who lived in Hong Kong, and inviting me to come and see them there. And lest I be accused of squandering my filial capital on the gambling tables of world travel, of becoming a black sheep, I made plans to go. Of course, I wanted to see them. It had been three years.

My flight into Hong Kong was late by two hours. An immigration official paged briskly through my passport, and with a quick flick of the wrist, stamped in it a two-week admission. Outside in the night a cosmopolitan web of buildings and highways rose around me. A thin Chinese man in a tattered undershirt looked up from his rest on a rattan cot outside a shop. Red double-decker buses rushed down the freeway.

Margaret, my father's younger sister, a Baptist missionary, lived in Kowloon Tong, a neighborhood on the mainland side. I made my way to her home and knocked on the door. We stayed up late exchanging family news. We didn't discuss my father's letter, but its themes, I think, hung over us.

Over the next week, we ventured into teeming, frenetic Hong Kong, where commercial energy pulsated along each alley and road. The crush of crowds on the street swept us forward, past Chinese teenagers squatting on street corners, shops where pictures of mustachioed ancestors presided over blood oranges and candles.

In a park, we watched as grandfathers clad in black performed their daily Tai Chi, swooping gracefully, right arms extended, wrists cocked, left arms held as if cradling a ball against their bellies. Back and forth they flowed, like waves, playing with energy, moving it through their bodies. Past them Chinese families strolled, chattering, happy.

We climbed the famous winding ladder-street and rode a ferry to the far side of the island. We immersed ourselves in the attractions of Hong Kong, a little at a loss for how to relate to each other. When last I'd seen my parents, I'd been an angrier young man, impatient, unable to talk about my emotional impasses. Now I felt calmer, more mature, but the context of my life was so different that it was difficult to know where to begin describing that life to them.

England's lease on Hong Kong was set to expire in 1997; the territory would then revert to the mainland Chinese Communists. People lived beneath a slowly expanding umbrella of anxiety about the future. "Human nature is not perfectible," Aunt Margaret declared while we were discussing Hong Kong's future at lunch with some friends. "We all have sin—you can't expect people to be ideal and only work for the collective interest! That's why the Communists in China haven't succeeded. And that's why Christ had to come."

I didn't tell her that I'd found in yoga something I'd been unable to find in our family's faith.

One of Margaret's Chinese friends asked me, perhaps grasping for a familiar touchstone, "What kind of meditation do you do? Is it Buddhist?"

"No, it comes from India. It's a kind of yoga."

Not long before, I'd read a short story about a cheerful Indian swami who visits a Western family and freaks out the tight-laced evangelical grandmother, until one night she sees him deep in meditation, levitating over his bed, and realizes he's a holy roller, too. On some level I guess I hoped for a similar home run, hoped that I could convey to them how we were both immersed in the spiritual life, simply coming at it from different angles.

That evening, waiting to be seated for dinner, we sat silently on a bench in a restaurant foyer. Suddenly, a man standing in front of us lost control. Falling smack over on the floor, he began writhing at our feet. Was he epileptic? Several people rushed to his aid, and the convulsions were brought under control. A little later an ambulance arrived and the paramedics rushed him away.

Watching this, for me at least, shattered some kind of spell: it was the urgent, breaking into the profane. The episode reminded me that life was not nice. Life was not tame. Life was unpredictable and dangerous and beautiful. Anything could happen. Couldn't my parents see that that was what I was embracing?

We parted a few days later and at the airport they asked, somewhat wistfully, "Will we see you back in the States soon?"

Time passes at different speeds for objects traveling at different rates. I was no longer, if I had ever been, traveling at the same speed as my parents. The choices I'd made, the changes I'd undergone, must have been difficult for them to understand. We held radically different views on the value of my time abroad. It reminded me of the Kurosawa film *Rashomon*: witnesses see the same event and yet tell wildly different versions of the story.

But of course, this was *my* story. I had to live it. And I had to make my own choices.

CHAPTER TWENTY-THREE

A young man with his blonde hair threaded in a ponytail loped down the aisle of the plane, checked his boarding pass, and then sat down in the seat across from me. He seemed vaguely familiar. He was eyeing me, too, as if something didn't make sense. Was he another margii?

It took a little time for me to process his features—dimpled chin, broad cheekbones, long face. Suddenly it hit me, and he seemed to make the connection in the same gradual fashion. A look of amazement swept across his face.

"Andy? Andy? I can't believe it!"

I hadn't seen Mark, a housemate from Helios, the housing cooperative in Austin, in over three years, and neither of us had known the other was in Asia. To be seated next to him on a flight out of Calcutta now bordered on the surreal.

Mark filled me in on what had happened to some of our mutual Helios friends. Allen and Michelle had broken up, Michelle taking off on a cross-country soul-searching ramble, and later making it big as a folk musician under the name Michelle Shocked. Yes, that Michelle Shocked. David had married, moved to Atlanta, and was working on the production staff at CNN. Pete was a corporate manager for a trucking firm. My friends were climbing the American career ladder, while I was engaged in something quite different. With a physical reminder of those Texas days now sitting across from me, I felt I was being asked to glance over my shoulder at the world I was leaving one last time.

As the plane arced across sprawling Calcutta, toward the Bay of Bengal and the shimmering rice fields of Thailand a couple of hours away, I let Mark in on my secret: I was on my way to the acharya training center in the Philippines.

"No way!" he said. "You're gonna become a monk? Wow....You nervous?"

"Not really, it's what I want to do."

I tried to explain to him what had happened over the last several years. Two years in Tokyo had seen the quashing of some demons, a surge in self-confidence, deepening spiritual practices clearing the cobwebs from my head. I had a great respect for many acharyas I'd worked with. I hoped somehow to be of service. And, of course, there was that ember of devotion glowing in my heart.

I smiled at Mark, and settled back in my seat.

I said goodbye to Mark in Bangkok, accepting his good wishes for my future. A week later I was on another plane, an overnight flight to Manila. From there I would catch a ferry to the island of Davao in the southern Philippines, where the training center was located. The plane's window visors were pulled down tightly since we would be flying east into an early sunrise. I tossed and turned in my seat. I was a little freaked out.

Going to training was a big step. *Did I have what it took to be an acharya?* Old complexes still called out to me, not wanting to be left behind. I knew there would be a long-term learning curve, and I also knew that I wouldn't be doing it alone. But the enormity of the move gave me pause. Fitfully, I fidgeted the late hours away.

In the morning, lurching to the back of the plane I squeezed into the tiny bathroom and splashed water on my face. I knew my decision was the right one. If I could just remain in touch with the spiritual spark that had brought me to this juncture, I would have nothing to worry about. So I sat, as I had so many times before, and would many times to come. I sat, and wrapped my arms around my confusion. And thanked God for the person I was becoming.

The plane touched down in Manila. I exited the airport lounge, ready to tangle with the usual suspects. A beggar approached, but unlike Indian beggars, this one was half-hearted, softer. He took 'no' for an answer. I had no money anyway, only bus fare. With directions for the AM office in my pocket, I jumped a bus headed for the inner-city neighborhood of Paco.

It was a moment of high political drama in the Philippines—January 1986—not long after the fall of Ferdinand Marcos. Corruption in the military had given way before priests and nuns kneeling in the path of government tanks, which in turn inspired workers, students and middle-class people to take to the streets in a genuine "people power" revolution. The presidential palace had been thrown open and Imelda Marcos' thousand and one pairs of shoes displayed to the masses, many of whom had no shoes at all. The most active Proutist group outside of India had played a role in the events that helped to topple Marcos, I was inspired to learn, agitating in the streets for change.

I got off the bus at Paz Street, then walked several more blocks, glancing at the slip of paper with the address in my hand, and at the numbers on the tree-shaded houses. Before me was the yoga center, a large walled house with a garden in front. I rang the bell and waited. The door swung open, revealing the face of an old friend, Dada P, the office secretary here. Surprised, he motioned me in. "Come in, come in. What are you doing here?"

"Oh, I'm thinking of spending some time in the south. You know, maybe Davao?"

A grin spread across his face. We embraced.

"It's about time," he laughed.

I would be in Paco for a week, waiting for the next ferry. In the mean time I needed to go to the market and buy some cloth, and then find a tailor to make my uniform. Trainees wore the saffron acharya uniform from day one at the training center. I wondered how this would feel.

I headed back to the main street where crowded jitneys—recycled U.S. army jeeps doubling as public transport—flashed by with their silver and red sideboards, plush buttoned ceilings and yellow plastic streamers flapping along in their wake. "Think God," a large sign on one proclaimed. I found a jitney heading for the market and slid inside. A statuette of Mother Mary sat planted on the dashboard while plastic silhouettes of naked girls flanked her, swinging back and forth in the cab as the driver negotiated the sprawling metropolitan traffic. At the market, I wended my way through endless stalls and finally found the shop Dada had recommended. After purchasing three yards of cloth, I explored a bit, wandering among the stalls and drinking in the warm and slow pace.

After India, the Philippines boasted the largest number of margiis. Hundreds attended weekly meditation and people were constantly dropping by the jagrti for meals or just to hang out. Filipinos, one man joked to me, were "born with a guitar in one hand and a cooking spoon in the other." It was a week of good food and friendly connection.

Soon, though, the day for departure arrived, and Dada drove me and another brother to the docks to catch the ferry. I would be traveling with a muscular, taciturn Nigerian named Ananta, also headed for the training center. Standing on a balcony over the main deck of the boat, we watched the shore pull away, its rocky outcroppings receding. There are 7017 islands in the Philippines republic, and our ferry would thread its way through a few of the largest ones. The trip to Mindanao would take three days.

Hearing calls from above, we looked up and were startled to see a group of ten men in orange-colored jumpsuits gripping the chain link of a fence.

"More traveling monks!" Ananta laughed. We shouted greetings over the thrum of the ship's engines. All of us were being ferried to our fates, they headed to the penal colony, we to the training center; their longing for physical freedom mirrored, perhaps, by Ananta and I yearning for freedom on another level.

The smoke of cigarettes in the boat's belly was unbearable and so we spent much of our time on deck. We also cooked our own food, bargaining with the cooks for vegetables, which we boiled on the ship's stove as these men watched over our shoulders.

Ananta was robust, tall and full of fire. We'd both been named Andrew by our respective parents. As he began to open up, he told me about his life in Lagos. He'd been a grade school teacher and enjoyed the work, but said he'd always longed for something more. Physically and temperamentally we were quite different, yet we became firm friends. I remember his laugh, deep and loud, racing up and down the scale like an arpeggio.

We passed Cebu on the evening of the second day. Ominous clouds dogged us. The wind picked up and the sea began to chop, while the sky darkened. Soon nature turned wild, the ocean recoiling in bursts of kinetic energy. As the boat bucked and rolled, we watched people drape themselves over the railing to retch into the sea. Queasy faces floated past. The crew scurried about assuring everyone that all would be fine.

While I was in Paco, an elderly Indian dada had told me about being lost at sea on these very deeps. Because of bad weather the captain had lost his bearings, his boat had turned around several times, and the passengers feared for their lives. Dada spoke of the intense relief of finally reaching safe harbor, mining the experience for spiritual metaphor. "It was like the freedom one feels," he told me, "when at long last, after many trials, one finds sanctuary."

Our boat remained on course, however, and the next morning dawned clear, the sea like glass. Passengers greeted each other heartily in the passageways. The boat slipped past Zamboanga, cock-fighting capital of the Philippines. We were nearing our destination. Wearily, on the evening of the third day, we docked at Davao.

On the pier several people waited to greet us. Reaching for our bags, three Filipinos led the way to a truck, and we piled in and proceeded down the faintly lit streets of Davao, toward the outskirts of town.

Turning onto a gravel road, one brother pointed to the top of a nearby bluff, from which lights cast a welcoming glow into the night. They were the lights of Davao Training Center, or *Praksinath Math*, our home for the foreseeable future.

Five buildings, cinder-block and wood, several with walls that only went waist-high, leaving them open to the breezes, stood on the two acres or so of land. A quarter-mile to the east was a rustic marketplace where shiny jitneys idled at the crossroads, and Spanish bread hung in wicker baskets in front of small rough shops. To the west lay forested land.

I sat at a picnic table, beneath the eaves of the main building that served as dining hall, reading a book from the center's library. The sun burned in the sky.

Ananta, who'd been exploring the grounds, sauntered over and lowered his muscular frame onto a seat. He looked at me and laughed. I laughed back. We were both a little giddy, unsure what to expect.

"Well," he said.

"Well, yourself."

Part of our uncertainty had to do with the sounds echoing out of the jungle from time to time. This morning in the meditation hall I'd folded my blanket on the floor and sat, looking forward to my first meditation here. Closing my eyes, I'd counted off the preliminary *japa* on my knuckle joints. A freshening breeze floated through the hall. I began to settle into a state of concentration, taut nerve cells in my brain relaxing. Yes, this was the stuff. My breathing slowed.

Deeper.

Quieter.

Ka-kkrang!!

I jerked upright and peered into the gloom.

When we heard the shots that morning, I'd flinched. But one of the Filipino trainees assured us that the fighting was miles away. He explained that Mindanao was home to two separate insurrectionary movements. One was fighting to form a Muslim republic on the island. The other, the New People's Army, military wing of the Philippines Communist Party, was especially strong. It wasn't uncommon to hear bullets whizzing by as NPA rebels traded shots with the military, or with the rapidly growing paramilitary groups.

Ananta and I expected to adjust to this, just as we hoped to adjust to the rigors of discipline. Despite the sense we had of Davao teetering on the edge of civilization, it seemed a good place to settle for a while.

Now the man in charge, the trainer, Dada Cidananda, ambled over. He looked the part of an Indian swami, tall and thin in his saffron tunic, with a long white beard and eyes set deeply in a face that beamed imperturbability. I could picture him meditating unflappably in high Himalayan snows.

"Is everything fine with you? Is there something you need?"

Cid, as we affectionately came to call him, was famous, at least among the hundreds of acharyas he'd trained. Fifteen years earlier, at Baba's direction, but without a peso, he'd opened this center on the outskirts of Davao, methodically constructing a complex of buildings and cottage industries (the manufacturing and sale of peanut candies, tofu, soap and shampoo brought in some income). Slowly he'd earned the support of the local people. A dogged determination bore him through years of struggle. He struck me as full of dynamism, but humble, a deeply intuitive man.

He explained to us the daily routine: meditation four times a day, study in the morning, work in the afternoon. We would be preparing for two separate exams, covering subjects from spiritual philosophy to elementary Sanskrit to Neo-Humanism to Conduct Rules. There was one phone, in the office. No TV. The kitchen was little more than a dark lean-to, with shelves for storing food at one end and an open fire-pit out of which flames had to be coaxed each morning to prepare meals. Books, and occasional newspapers, were available but for the period of our training, we would live apart from the world.

Ananta and I glanced at each other. Though most of the trainees were in their twenties, the typical distractions of a young person were absent here. No alcohol, tobacco, or drugs. No extensive wardrobe, or battery of personal grooming products. No electronics. No Mustangs or Volvos. No discretionary income, at all.

And there was that little matter of the vow of celibacy. Women were to be seen as sisters, men as brothers, and the energy of any residual sexual fascination would have to be redirected. I was OK with that. Any thoughts of former crushes, of Maria in Tokyo, I felt sure, would fade in this new environment. For three years I'd lived among monks, observed how they embraced this commitment. Now it was my turn.

And in the coming months Cid would remind us that it was attachment, not love, we were working to curtail: "Strive to perceive in everything the curve of underlying spirit, interact with each person as an expression of the divine, and love that divine spark." He added,

"And be prepared to let go of whatever distracts you from that commitment."

A clothesline ran between the buildings where we sat, on which this morning I had hung my *laungota*, or yogic underwear, out to dry. Dada Cid zeroed in on it. "Whose is this?"

"It's mine, Dada-ji."

A rip, which was spreading into a large hole, ran across the middle of my yogic shorts. Since it occurred where the cloth draped around the back of the body, and didn't impede function, if function was the right word, I'd decided with my usual frugality to wear it in this state as long as I could. I could have borrowed needle and thread and stitched it up. But, I thought, what's the difference?

He turned to me. "Why are you wearing this? Either sew it up or get a new one."

"But, Dada, it doesn't make any difference. No one can see it. It's underwear."

"If no one can see it, how is it that I'm seeing it right now?"

Good point. A little embarrassed, I nevertheless appreciated his implicit emphasis: No ragged edges. A monk's life must be clear-cut, a spirituality grounded in practicality. It was all about the way one did things.

"I'll mend it, Dada."

He smiled. "Use your time here wisely." Then he stood up. "And don't think too much." And he was gone into the office.

I didn't have time to think much.

That weekend we prepared food to distribute in the barrio. In the low clapboard kitchen I jostled elbows with other trainees, many of them Filipinos, their long black hair tumbling down their backs, as we peeled root vegetables, which we tossed into a huge cooking pot along with rice, shredded coconut, and sugar. Among the seventy or so people here—thirty male trainees, ten female trainees (who lived in another house several miles away and came to the center for classes during the day), the orphans in the children's home, and staff—the majority were Filipino. My companions expressed themselves in a complicated combination of consonants and unexpected diphthongs, the Visayan language, that seemed designed for good-natured teasing and banter. They glanced at me curiously, but amiably.

When we'd finished cooking, we poured the still-bubbling *lugao* into small containers, hauled these onto the back of the center's rickety pickup truck, and shuddered out onto the highway. This was my first real daytime view of the city. As we drove through the long winding side streets of Davao, kids tugged at their mothers' sleeves, pointing, "Look, ma, the yoga people!"

The truck made a sharp right and headed down to the docks. The sea, its briny foam specked with paper cups and food wrappers, sloshed noisily against the frame of the pier. We drove onto the beach where rows of dilapidated shacks on stilts formed a community beneath a wall of swaying coconut trees. As we disembarked, young kids who had been playing kick-the-can began trailing us across the sand. Suddenly, hundreds of children were streaming out from the village, cartwheeling from the soccer field to the beach, converging on our truck.

Children of all ages and sizes lined up, most of them in ragged shorts and T-shirts, barefoot and grinning, clutching pot, bowl, or glass, and spoon. A small boy in a grimy shirt with the cartoon dog Pluto stenciled on the front ran up to stare at Ananta and me, then darted back behind the safety of his big brother's legs.

It was great. I felt like Santa Claus, a foreign spectacle, a good man. The kids loaded up on sweet rice, and we all lounged on the beach. The sea crept closer to our party, as the sun inched toward the horizon. One brother had brought along a guitar, and he curled the fingers of his left hand around the strings, languidly picking out a Filipino folk song, the gentle rhythm echoing out across the furrows of sand.

On the far side of the sky the moon appeared, waning toward a quarter of its original shape, though the whole could be perceived in milky outline, like a half-empty vessel spilled out, waiting to be filled again.

CHAPTER TWENTY-FOUR

A voice pierced the silence, the 4:40 a.m. wakeup call. I bolted upright in the darkness and stumbled to the bathhouse to splash cold water over my body. The morning stars shone faintly in the sky; on the horizon lay a hint of color. Silently, we wrapped ourselves in blankets to sit for sadhana. In the pale light, the thirty or so blanketed bodies were tiny mountains rising from the floor.

A few minutes before seven, I stretched and looked around. I'd been meditating for an hour and a half, and my mind felt clear. I stood, shook off my blanket, and ambled over to the clearing in front of the main hall to hear the announcements. "We need more firewood." "Don't lose the knives after cooking—keep them in the proper place." The monitor read out the weekly duties. "K will be kitchen-in-charge. D, cleaning-in-charge." There were some groans.

Afterwards we sat at a long picnic table for breakfast. A shelf of white rice sat on my plate, next to a heap of skinny green beans, slightly buried by a few stir-fried tomatoes. I frowned as I picked up my fork. After a week, I was bored with the food here already. The challenges of the place were beginning to become apparent. Still, my meditation was good.

We slept on sleeping mats on the floor of the main building in a large open space. Privacy was at a premium. Mornings, I heard the Italian brother coughing and wheezing across the room, his allergies giving him hell. And the Argentine, Ras Mohan, in the corner, all his scraps of paper and odd items of clothing scattered around him. He was the messiest person I'd ever seen; junk seemed to pull around him like electrons to a nucleus.

A young Nigerian slept on my other side, tall and muscular as a welterweight boxer, often snoring and snorting like a bull. The first time we'd met, Prakash had unburdened himself to me, telling me about the slights he'd felt at the hands of various people. He spoke in rapid-fire cadences, with a constitutional anger that meditation seemed to have done little to blunt. Later, he thought better of his openness, perhaps thinking I would use his confessions against him, and he began to pick quarrels. He would spend the next year oscillating between excitable friendship and sullen resentment toward me.

Fortunately, there were also trainees like Santosa. This young man, whose name meant 'mental contentment,' hailed from Bali, and the energy of that lush Pacific island, of its *wayang kulit* shadow puppet creativity, seemed to radiate from him. Beneath neatly trimmed black hair, his dark eyes sparkled with intelligence, and his voice rang out like music. He was self-possessed, often smiling or joking, and moved unobtrusively, reminding me of one of those figures in a Chinese landscape painting, tucked in to the cleft of a mountain pass, dwarfed by the immense wildness and beauty of nature around him, but definitely a part of it all.

If most of us in Davao were striving to smooth out rough edges, the bramble bushes of our egos tangling with and scratching those around us, Santosa seemed beyond many of these personal dramas. He was one of those rare people who seemed to have done their personal work already, born into this world carefree. As I struggled to find my footing, his friendship, a kind word here and there, sustained me.

Dada Cid had long ago decided that one way to immerse his trainees in good clean living was through karma yoga. Otherwise known as grunt work. Spirituality, Cid professed, was to be found in the generation of sweat. The buildings at the training center had been constructed by trainees, and the place was constantly expanding. The sequence of development seemed haphazard, though, and some had stood half-completed for years. Cid wanted us to work on finishing some of these.

My work partner was a tall, slightly aloof Italian. He pointed out the wooden box we would use to transport sand and rocks to the construction site. Hefting the box by parallel poles extending along either side of it, we hobbled along, our triceps straining. We dumped our load next to the skeleton of the new building, while another brother ripped open a fifty-pound sack of concrete mix and poured it out, leaping back from the choking swirl of chalky dust that billowed from the heap.

The Italian and I fell into conversation as we mixed sand with concrete. We seemed to have a lot in common. Back in Italy, he told me, he'd entered the priesthood.

"What happened?"

He looked down for a moment, thoughtful. "The priesthood, it doesn't fill me with, how you say, the presence of God. I have faith, you know, but not the experience of God."

I nodded and watched as a Filipino trainee, dangling from the tangle of scaffolding and grinning, hoisted buckets to the top and dumped the mixture into cast molds to form foundation pillars.

Leaning on my shovel, I thought back to the sultry summer I'd dug ditches with a construction firm in Arlington, building a sprinkler system for a new golf course on the edge of town. That, too, had been hard work, and my muscles had bulged by the end of the summer, but wage labor in suburbia had quickly gotten old. Here in Davao, though no one had signed up to learn to mix concrete, the emphasis on hard practical work was refreshing, at least for a while; it added to the sense of brotherhood we were developing.

And there were moments of transcendence. One morning, eight of us contemplated building a restraining wall for a slowly eroding section of the campus overlooking the road. It was a big project, probably several days of work.

We set to it. It was a hot day, and cloudless. Santosa serenaded us with a Balinese folk song, his soft quavering voice offsetting the scraping sound of our shovels. Something else hung in the air, too, as work got under way: a sense of pushing ourselves beyond our usual limits.

After a while I glanced at Ananta. Leaning on his shovel, he cleared his throat, and peered at Prakash. Prakash punched me on the arm, a little harder than necessary. The Italian pulled a long drag from a bottle of water. A smile slowly appeared on each of our faces, evidence of some goofy collective high. In an intuitive flash, we sensed that we might finish the project in a single day.

At lunchtime, the monitor's whistle blew from up the hill. We shrugged and continued working. There seemed to be all the time in the world, all kinds of time, and no need to worry about anything.

Our rhythms moved to a higher pitch. Scrape, scrape. Shovel, shovel. Muscles straining, sweat flying, adrenalin pumping, we were John Henrys on the railroad. In this space of possibility we'd entered, our determination, it seemed, could have no other end. We were *motivated*.

The sun spun down in the sky. And, at five in the afternoon, Santosa reached out and laid the final brick on the wall. Everyone let out a cheer and plopped to the ground, too tired to do anything but sit and bask in satisfaction. After half an hour we staggered, muscles aching, to a shower, a quick meditation, and the lunch that had been kept covered for us.

"Man," Ananta said as we tucked in to our food. "I feel like we really did something today, you know?"

We were exhausted. But it was a wonderful tiredness, a kinetic tiredness, in which, like after a long hard swim, the seeds of renewed strength were sown.

In the West, the standard for monastic life has always been St. Benedict's rule: poverty, celibacy, and obedience. In Greek the rule is called *tremon*, from which the word trellis comes. Something to grow on. The difficulties of such a life, both in Benedict's fifth century CE, and now, are apparent, and clearly not for everyone. Benedict miraculously survived a poisoning attempt made by his first band of monks who grumbled over his strict demands. He went on to found twelve monasteries, which he spent the rest of his life directing. He noted that the monastic community is designed to absorb all the energies—physical, psychic and spiritual—of its members "whose individual perfection lay in the perfecting of the life of the whole."

"The abbot must recognize the difficulty of his position," Benedict wrote, "to care for and guide the spiritual development of many different characters. One must be led by friendliness, another by sharp rebukes, another by persuasion."

Like Benedict's abbot, Dada Cid was responsible for guiding and disciplining us, for hammering out our rough edges, melding individual energies into a strong collective force. For the most part he did this admirably.

Occasionally, though, young men arrived claiming they wanted to become monks who clearly were not suited for acharya life. Perhaps they came to work off a certain delinquent energy. Thomas Merton described such individuals who arrive at monastic life with "no sense of what it means to live in community, who were individualistic, from dysfunctional families, wanting to be alone." Many of us fit this bill, but we were, for the most part, able to adjust. If someone couldn't Dada Cid usually perceived it early on and suggested that the training center was not the place for them. Other times, perhaps tuning in to some psychic knot that cried out to be untied, he agreed to let them stay, and allowed things to play out.

Narayan, a new Filipino trainee, was said to be sneaking out at night to meet girls in the city. But his interactions with Prakash were what really stirred things up. The two took an immediate disliking to each other. Both were young and hardheaded, and they circled each other like alpha dogs, bristling whenever their paths crossed.

One evening I overheard an argument on the porch. "Man, you think you're something."

"You… you'd better watch your step." Then the voices died away. Something was up between those two.

The next morning after breakfast a few of us were upstairs preparing for class. Narayan rounded the corner, spied Prakash in the main room, and leapt. They tussled, saffron and white cloth fluttering. Prakash aimed a punch at Narayan, who responded in kind, and then fell back, scuffing with his foot at the floor. An object skittered away.

I was stunned. The new brother had lunged at Prakash with a knife, though he hadn't stabbed him, and mostly seemed to have used it as a bluff. Dada Cid, somehow aware of the fracas, came charging up the stairs and chastised them both. Prakash brushed himself off, glanced around at the rest of us, and smirked.

"You," Dada said to Prakash. "Go downstairs."

"And you," he said to Narayan, his voice rising in disbelief. "You used a knife?" Cid expelled the boy straightaway. Perhaps those knots had had enough untying for now.

We discussed the incident for days. The sisters, who joined us for lunch, grilled us for the details. Narayan had never really made a commitment to this way of life, someone noted; he hadn't taken his sadhana seriously. Another person remarked that not everyone who came here was suited to become an acharya. It was true. Statistically speaking, more than a third of us would not see the training through.

Then someone brought up the story of Kalicharan, the first person to whom Baba had taught meditation. A notorious criminal, he'd tried to rob Baba one night on a lonely road on the outskirts of Calcutta. But like Saul on the road to Damascus, in Baba's presence his life was turned upside down, or rather, right side up. I loved that story, its message of human frailty and potential for redemption, the idea that we were all bound together in a common humanity both by our weakness and a desire for transcendence.

The first initiate had been a criminal. What could we take from this? Perhaps that this was a path that attracted all sorts, including folks who might have heavy karma to work through. Who were we to judge anyone? If you were sincere (and Narayan, Dada seemed to have determined, was not, at least at this point in time), there was still a place for you at this table. Maybe Narayan would be back.

Beyond that, the lesson seemed to be that you might not like somebody, but you had to learn to love them. A person bugged you, drove you to distraction, and you could either obsess until you began to take on those qualities yourself, or be patient. Be patient and love them. Take note of the qualities in yourself that they set astir like a hornet's nest.

Sartre wrote that hell is other people. A yogic take would spin it differently: Difficult people are your teachers.

And anyone, really, could be difficult. The revolving constellations of friendship among the trainees shifted over time as dramatically as each of us was changing individually. Cliques formed. Resentments brewed. We were all pretty young, stumbling along the bumpy borderline that separated young adults from men. That was part of the equation. But I also think many of the struggles we faced involved the intense expression of *samskara*, or karmic reaction, each of us meeting our limitations head on in an environment with thirty other determined young men doing deep meditation and undergoing their own personal struggles. All of us working to relax the tight grip of ego.

In ordinary life, our egos waltzed us through the world, engaged us in amusing activities, tugged us toward agreeable others, or invoked an aversion to fools. The mystical path saw this worldly understanding of ego as incomplete. Here, the aim was: not I, but God through me.

Of course, it would be simplistic to say that ego was bad and non-ego good. Ego was a part of us, always there, useful in certain ways. What we were discovering was that there were deeper layers of self upon which we could draw, quieter, more soulful ways of being into which we might settle. When we weren't driving each other crazy.

The round of days rolled on. Monsoon rains once again blew in from the deeps. Each day a cycle renewed itself. Sometimes the dull grip of boredom seized us. But some new project, new trainee arrival, or deep meditation always broke the spell. A few trainees began to teach in one of the schools AM oversaw in town.

Dada Cid returned from a trip to India. We lined up to greet him, like grandkids welcoming home a grandfather. Dada bore gifts for all the orphanage kids—mostly new clothes. Affection shone in his eyes as each little child came forward to claim their present. We looked on with avuncular pleasure.

It was a relaxed day, and everyone gathered around the kitchen, laughing and talking. We slipped root vegetables from the pantry into the fire pit for roasting, testing them with knives, then carried them outside, sliding off the sheath of skin and blowing on the steaming yellowish tubers to cool them. They were very sweet.

CHAPTER TWENTY-FIVE

Be accustomed to live a hard and industrious life.
—Conduct Rules

Months passed. Most mornings before I got up I sprawled on my back, tugging a rough blanket over my feet, twisting my body to one side to avoid a knot in the hard planked floor. The monitor's whistle would blow in a few minutes and I wanted to squeeze in a few more delicious moments of sleep.

Exams were coming up, but I couldn't seem to concentrate, to memorize any of the conduct rules. I always seemed to be tired. A visiting acharya offered me Vitamin B tablets, said they were good for the brain. Prakash, ever the critic, scoffed: "He's taking a pill to improve his memory!"

The heat and the rain, the daily grind of study, the personality clashes, a kind of physical lassitude—lately, things had been piling up and getting me down. Occasionally all was swept away in a flood of ecstasy. But only occasionally.

Day after sticky day we sat down at the dining table to tedious sameness: rice three times a day, and only a slight variation on the theme of stir-fried vegetables. A sympathizer who managed a plantation had hauled over a truckload of bananas, but how many bananas could a person eat? We lived on an island renowned for fruit—luscious papaya, starfruit, custard apple, and mangosteen—but since there were so many of us, the fruits we collected were first offered to the sisters, and the remainder turned into mushy fruit salad. We had enough to eat, but not enough that was interesting to eat.

We'd been studying a *sutra* that should have held comfort for me: *An obstacle is that helping force which establishes one confronted by it in the goal.* Although I appreciated the idea of *the helping force*— that the spiritual path was littered with obstacles but also with a hidden energy, and that overcoming these obstacles zipped you along the path— I didn't feel helped. Not at the moment, anyway.

I knew I was expected to be strong, to do the Tantric thing, but I didn't always feel that way. Sometimes I felt vulnerable. Not surprisingly, this began to surface in the training center, and so sometimes my mantra, in compensation, became 'I want, I want, I want.'

One Sunday a celebration was held to mark the graduation of some of the older trainees. There were speeches, and a feast of special food—delicately fried blocks of tofu with soy sauce and sesame, greens with ginger, sweet rice. Maybe it had to do with the struggles I was facing. Maybe it was the unusually appealing food situation. Or maybe I was supposed to learn something the hard way. But on this day desire surged against my skillfully constructed dam of control and rose precariously over the floodplain of my appetites. I shoveled the food in, eating way too much.

Santosa was sitting across from me, telling the story of how, when he was a student attending university in Bali, he sometimes had only one meal a day. And how he learned to be satisfied with that. Good old Santosa. He watched me go for a few moments. "Hey," he said, smiling, "a little restraint."

I nodded, but it was too late anyway. Pushing heavily away from the table, I plodded upstairs. A friend was sitting on a bench, and hailed me, "Hey, bro, you want some papaya?"

"Umm, sure." Who knew when I might get some papaya again? Besides, wasn't it good for digestion?

In another room, the offer was made, "Biscuit?"

"OK." I'd been working hard, I thought, I deserved a few biscuits.

Now my digestion was creaking. Too much, too much. I had to get out, to go for a walk. I left the dorm and strolled toward the forest. The merciless sun was beating down, the walk not helping, and I felt sick. Why, oh why, had I eaten so much? Other trainees passed by, asking, "How's it going?" I grunted. Prakash loped by and smirked, as if he knew what was happening inside of me.

Homer had Odysseus remark, "Is there nothing more doglike than this hateful belly? It always arouses us, even at the height of anguish." Here I was, face to face with my own weakness, nowhere to hide. I went to my room and lay my rebellious body down.

Several days later during class, Dada Cid reproved me out of the blue.

"You are the greediest one here!"

I stared at him. He couldn't have known about my binge. But he'd pegged me, all right. I did have a tendency toward self-indulgence, mostly as a way to fill the hole that had been in me since I was young.

The discipline here was beginning to make a dent in this, substituting a spiritual goal for physical indulgence, just as fasting had done when Indian Dada introduced it to me in Bangkok. But it would take time.

My guess is that Cid was simply doing what he did, picking up intuitively on the struggles of his trainees and trying to steer us in the right direction. His insight amazed me. I felt, not confronted, but relieved.

"You're right, Dada."

When it came to reproofs from Dada Cid I was able to put my ego aside. How could I feel ashamed in the presence of someone who clearly pointed out my faults with an eye toward helping me rectify them? Through all our mistakes as young and inexperienced trainees, Dada was patient. He didn't dwell on my error, and moved on to another topic. But somehow his words had done their work. I stood corrected.

Can I say that after some time the flames of desire began to sputter and subside to a reasonable height? That was the ideal. Only after struggling with desire, shadowing its course, understanding where it led, could I put it aside. Whether or not I could always control my passions, I was beginning to discover that monastic life was not about peace and quiet, not about passive retreat. It was, at times, about facing the raging compulsions within, the hundred and one pettinesses, slights and jealousies, embracing them, and then melting them into a bonfire of vanities fueled by our practices and our determination.

Kazantzakis had something to say on what perhaps was a similar matter. "God is fire, and you must walk on it, dance on it. At that moment the fire will become cool water. But until you reach that point, my Lord, what agony!"

As it turns out, all the trainees were, to a lesser or greater degree, obsessed with food.

Most of us had little caches of bread or cookies we'd received while asking for food donations in the marketplace. For the most part, nobody dissented with the actual existence of, or even necessity of what we called, with a touch of irony, *black food*. But distribution was another matter. My Italian friend said that since we were here to learn to live collectively, black food should be shared equally. Prakash, not surprisingly, thought there was nothing wrong with an individual reward for hard work, and since the marketing duties were rotated, everyone had a chance to receive treats.

Was it every man for himself? Or could we move toward a more egalitarian, perhaps more Proutist, model of sharing? This tension underlay our table manners.

A new trend also marked this period: the construction of little lockers in which to store our goodies. I think Prakash built the first one from scraps of wood left lying around. The idea took off, and soon most of the trainees had gleefully, if sheepishly, cobbled together small birdhouse boxes. In the evenings we sat around, popped open our stashes, had a snack and chatted about the day. But since black food was technically prohibited, these little boxes also held the taint of the illegitimate.

Dada Cid was traveling. Dada PR, an imposing American acharya, was sitting in as trainer *pro tem*. Cid had rarely come up to our sleeping quarters. I suspect he didn't actually care that much about black food. But PR did. Perhaps wanting to acquaint himself fully with the center's layout, he ventured upstairs one day. Noticing the row of wobbly little lockers perched above our beds, he opened one up.

I glanced at Ananta. What would Dada say?

As their utility dawned on him, PR began to fume. "What is this? Where is your discipline? What are you here for?"

PR ordered the boxes destroyed. We complied with a mixture of regret and perhaps relief, bearing our creations to the second story balcony and tossing them off into the courtyard. They arced through the air as if in slow motion, and then, hitting the ground, splintered, imploding like houses laid flat by a tornado, and lay in a heap. The staff carpenter, a simple Filipino man, stood by and looked on with interest.

Afterward, he gathered the wood together for one of his projects.

Upon returning from his trip, Cid decided it was time to rotate the positions of responsibility among the trainees, something he did occasionally. I had some vague expectation that I would be made storekeeper, he who kept his eye on the provisions of food and distributed them to the cooks. I wouldn't mind doing that.

One day Dada turned to me, "I have something special in mind for you."

I smiled. He smiled.

"Not storekeeper," he said.

The next day he announced: "A. will be the new monitor."

Prakash gave a low whistle. The monitor oversaw the training center's routine, and made sure everybody followed it. He wielded some power, and had to be something of a badass to make sure people toed the line. The position required managerial grit. I'd heard tales about monitors at the training center in Sweden—how exacting they were, especially those punctilious Germans—and how much they clashed everyone out.

Of course, here in the laid-back Pacific, things moved at a different pace. Nevertheless, discipline was supposed to be the bedrock of our lives, and the monitor was charged with enforcing this. Dada Cid was in charge, of course, but he relegated a lot of authority to the monitor. Once again, it seemed, someone had seen in me something I had not seen in myself. I was pleased, but a little worried. How would I manage it?

I began by drawing up the weekly roster, neatly ruling off the sheet of paper with ruler and pencil, striving for some kind of parity. Let's see, K will do the cooking, JM the marketing. Who'll clean the bathrooms? Each morning a volley of complaints and counter-complaints followed announcements, and it was my duty as monitor to sort them all out. "He didn't clean the pots and pans!" Yes, yes, O.K. Things seemed to be going all right.

One day I watched from across the campus as Ananta returned from a shift of making tofu. SB, a short, intense Filipino, planted himself in Ananta's path. Words were exchanged. Bristling with anger, SB thrust his chest into the other man's body. Then Ananta swung forward and awkwardly shoved SB. There they stood, inches apart, glaring.

Who knew what it was about? Endless opportunities existed for treading on toes, poking into personal spaces. Ananta could be stubborn, and I knew SB harbored an irrational resentment of the non-Filipinos here. But it was my responsibility to try to restore order. Ananta had stomped away, so I went down to speak with SB.

I wanted to be fair. How can we work this out? SB angrily muttered his complaint, as if he was certain nothing would ever be changed, something about how Ananta had misjudged some tofu technicality. He bumped my shoulder and began to barge away, but I walked alongside him, murmuring 'uh-huh' sounds to signal I was paying attention. My softness began to penetrate his defenses. It seems he was also upset about his duties for that week, something I could do something about. He calmed down.

Baba quoted the Buddha, *If someone is angry, you must win him over by a cool temper. If someone is dishonest, win him over by your honesty. Change a miser by spending something on him.* It was good advice, as usual. Clash between trainees was bound to happen. I couldn't prevent it (in fact preventing it might have been counterproductive), but I could help to channel the energies a little. This was my style, and sometimes it worked.

I couldn't always take this approach, however, and perhaps Cid had appointed me monitor in order to bring out another side of me, like turning over a mattress so all sides received equal pressure.

The arrival of monsoon season occasioned a spate of sleeping in, people disappearing into their blankets like burrows, striving to be cozy on the cold and blustery mornings. Concerned about this breach, we collectively decided on a new rule: those who did not get up at five for meditation would have to skip breakfast.

The next morning, I checked the roster. K, a Filipino, had slept in. I duly noted it and at breakfast announced he would not be served.

"It's the rule," I said, a little defensively.

K glared at me, sitting stiffly at the table as everyone else was served. I felt uneasy. Suddenly, another Filipino brother picked up his own full plate, slid it across to K, and without a word got up and walked away.

Prakash laughed, watching to see what would happen next.

I said nothing, though I was a little taken aback. Should I take this plate away, too? Hold fast to the rule-setting paradigm of a Westerner, while these brothers were acting with the nurturing instincts of family members, the sentimentality of Filipinos, something I admired? Such hardness was against my nature.

What would I do?

CHAPTER TWENTY-SIX

Davao was, for most of the year, a warm and sun-drenched place. Palm coconut and jackfruit trees towered overhead; the sound of the ocean surf could be heard not far away. It seemed an unlikely setting for the beginning of so much physical difficulty.

Even in Tokyo, my health had not been great. Endless belching as my digestive system struggled to make sense of its environment had not endeared me to the others in the PROUT office. Maybe it was because I'd been eating different food, living in a colder climate, or sitting at a desk most of the day. Maybe Calcutta's undrinkable water had taken its toll. All I knew was that if things were freeing up for me on one level, physically life was becoming more complicated.

Here in Davao, the intestinal problems continued. I practiced the *utksepa mudra*, an asana aimed at stimulating the elimination system, clasping my knees to my chest and flinging them out again. But it didn't always help. My health seemed to be stagnating.

One evening, upon returning from marketing, I leapt down from the back of the truck and as my feet touched the ground a razor-sharp pain shot up my leg. Without my noticing, my left foot had swollen up like a balloon to twice its normal size. I crumpled to the ground.

Two brothers supported me as I hobbled up the stairs. This was no simple insect bite, but a serious infection. I was transferred to a bed in the office downstairs so that I wouldn't have so far to go to the bathroom, but as it was I could barely get out of bed.

For a few days I lay there, staring at my foot puffed up like an obese adder. One of the children's home kids came in to visit me. "Eet ees veerry beeeg, Dada!" he joked.

When it became apparent that the swelling would not reduce on its own, Valmiki, my old friend from Malaysia who had also recently arrived for training, drove me to the nearby public hospital.

Val pushed me in a wheelchair down a long corridor through the middle of an ongoing construction project where flakes of plaster and dust billowed into the passageway and settled on my swathed ankle. Finally we made it through the gauntlet of carpenters with their easygoing banter and the sounds of pounding nails and power saws, to the waiting room where I reached down and brushed the debris from my leg.

Fifty people perched on plastic chairs, each cradling their complaint. From the row behind, I heard patients muttering that many of the medical supplies had been siphoned off to a U.S. naval hospital at another city. "All the good medicine goes there, lah, and we get stuck with the leftovers." This may have been idle gossip, but it seemed clear the facility was struggling. Harried nurses rushed by, and occasionally someone was called in for an exam. The high-speed pitch of power saws in the next wing whined on. Finally I met with a doctor who changed the dressing on my foot and prescribed antibiotics, but no name was ever given to my condition, no real explanation to help me make sense of it.

For the next four weeks I lay on my back, reading, listening to the chatter of life outside the office walls, or to the occasional sound of gunfire in the distance. Sometimes I dragged myself outside to drink in a different vista. Occasionally a visitor came bearing a gift of fried bananas. I meditated propped up against a pillow in bed. On top of the infection, during this period I lost an amazing amount of weight—40 pounds—down from 150 to 110. Where did it all go? I was practicing non-accumulation, but this was ridiculous. I looked like a stick figure.

While recuperating in the office, I watched life go on in the sultry heat. Sometimes when I woke it was with a pounding headache and a weakness in my limbs that hinted that my energy had been sapped centrifugally. I missed more morning meetings. Eventually, since I couldn't keep up with my responsibilities, Dada appointed Ananta to be monitor.

That, as I said, was the beginning. Though the swelling receded, the strange infection of my left foot seemed to set the stage, for afterwards, I was hit by a series of even more debilitating illnesses. Davao was the pivotal point in my seven year sojourn in Asia, bisecting the two views of myself, old and new, ordinary person and monk. In Davao, my spiritual life gelled into solidity. But it was also the beginning of a physical breakdown, the gradual sinking of my body into chronic illness.

Trying to make sense of it all, I recalled Dada Dharma in Japan telling me that when he was a young acharya he'd developed terrible eczema. He'd just had to ride it out, he said, see it as a spiritual test. "Have patience," he told me. "Things will work out. Your karma will work itself out."

Really, everything depended on one's outlook. According to Tantric philosophy, one's *samskara* had to be undergone, which could involve a lot of pain. How you dealt with that pain, however, was another matter; there was a distinct difference between pain and suffering. I remembered the struggles I'd had in Calcutta and my realizations about how to deal lightly with them. Ideally, spiritual practices put you in good stead, kept you in a blissful state, helped you to cope. And when they didn't, Yogananda's adage was helpful: "Pain is a prod to remembrance. If joy were ceaseless here, would man ever desire more?" Pain had meaning in its moving us to look for answers beyond the mundane.

And really, despite the pain, in a single moment everything could change. Listening to a brother who had come to visit me describe Baba's commitment to uplifting humanity, my mind broke free from its fumbling preoccupations with the lapses of my body, as if it had been tethered by straps to the earth which were now cut.

I'd been given to worrying too much. In these sweet moments of pausing my anxieties dispersed. My ego—rough guide, easily detoured—relaxed, and another state of being floated in. Beautiful. Why couldn't it be this way all the time?

Slowly the infection cleared. And while in bed, I heard about changes taking place at the training center. Income from the cottage industries, along with donations from former trainees, were precipitating some new developments. Dada had long had a vision of building a coconut-oil processing co-op. Now he began to act on it. A machine shop was set up on the back lot.

The coconut plant was developed as part of a network of commercial products under the Lotus label distributed by AM in the Philippines. Based on appropriate technology, it was designed to employ large numbers of impoverished villagers. This was a good place for it, as the Philippines were number one in world coconut production. For a time, copra and coconut oil rolled off that back lot, and a good price was paid to local farmers. Later, as the business developed, an offset printing press was acquired, and a charitable foundation was set up to construct houses for nearby squatter families.

I watched all this growth, impressed with Dada's ability to realize his vision. But I wouldn't be around much longer to see what else happened. After a year in Davao, having passed the two exams, done a lot of deep meditation, fallen sick and recovered somewhat, I now set out with my classmates to do Special Training. This was the culmination of our time here, a week of intense practices modeled after the lives of renunciate monks in India. The night before we began, we gathered in Dada Cid's office. He outlined what to expect.

"You will wear only two pieces of white cloth. No soap, comb, toothbrush, anything of that nature." We all smiled, expectant. "You will not speak for one week. You may go to the market with a small clay pot and silently ask for donations of food. Receive it gratefully and say nothing. Then bring back whatever you receive, prepare it over a small fire, and have your one meal per day."

Ananta and I smiled at each other. Having been through so much together since that ferry ride down from Manila a year ago, we were almost done; almost acharyas!

The next day dawned bright. A week of silence stretched before us like a great plain to be traversed. We stayed in a half-finished building away from the main campus, and at noon we spread out to try for some food, in places we knew. We were not to speak, although we could explain what we were doing if someone asked. I moved from shop to shop, standing in front of the shopkeepers with my bowl extended, a little embarrassed. Most of them were familiar with the ritual and glad to give a little something. I peered over to see what Ananta had received. An avocado!

Coming back from the market, I gathered twigs and branches, and lit one of my matches. The fire caught, though the wind threatened to blow out the flame, and I tried to keep my body between it and the fire. Slowly, the flames grew, and I placed my small clay pot into a little valley between pieces of wood. The earthen container soon became streaked with black smudges as my rice, green vegetables, and carrots simmered. Then I thoroughly enjoyed my one simple meal of the day.

It was not easy to go for a week without speaking. I wanted to compare notes with the others. But, as with the daily hour-long silences that were part of the regular training center routine, the practice grew on me. Existing in these broader landscapes of silence allowed an awareness of my energies to bubble up in the momentarily clear pool of my mind, the silt of my desires to settle and become clear. I was reminded that I often took for granted the way I acted, too rarely challenged the acquisitive stance of "What's in it for me?"

And so I resolved to enter more deeply into an understanding of what my desires were and how I expressed them. Within the silence I began to find more depth, discovering a delicious sense of freedom, of self-containment. It was an amazing thing.

Each afternoon, we worked, clearing brush from the perimeter of the training center. To communicate with each other, we pointed and gestured, or just took initiative, plunging into the ravine along the road, dragging old bushes and dying branches to a big pile, yanking weeds, smoothing out the rough earth.

Nights we slept wrapped in thin blankets on the ground. There was freedom in this way of life—no possessions to worry about, our days stretched out predictably before us. Tired from the semi-fasting of one meal a day, I slept part of each afternoon. But mornings I woke early and sank into a satisfying two hours of sadhana.

Sometimes I exchanged glances with Ananta or Valmiki or even Prakash. I saw the same sense of joy reflected in their eyes. Once again, the daily grind was subverted through the charm of our commitment to practice.

Once again the world became suffused with meaning.

CHAPTER TWENTY-SEVEN

Out beyond the curve of the bay we could see the steel prows of cargo ships anchored at sea. From the deck of one ship a blue flame flared against the gray sky. Gulls wheeled overhead, and breakers rolled onto the shore. A few Chinese couples strolled by on the beach, holding hands. Emerging from the surf, Prakash shook his Afro, slinging drops of seawater that refracted against the setting sun.

Not long before, on the eve of our graduation ceremony in Davao, a group of us had been shepherded to the tailor's to be fitted for new uniforms. The tailor stretched his measuring tape along the folds and lengths of our torsos, making a few notations in his notebook. The next day he brought out some orange cloth he'd fashioned to our bodies. The tunics seemed ill-fitting, but perhaps that was simply because of their newness. Dressed in our new saffron gowns, we took our places with the other acharyas in the meditation hall that evening. Did I imagine it, or had there been a slight stir when we entered? There *was* something different about us.

Now I was bobbing in the blue waters of Singapore's Johor Straits, watching Prakash and Valmiki bodysurf as they crashed into the breakers and rode them to shore. Our future lay uncharted before us. An acharya, I mused, was always moving, testing his or her limits, trusting in something beyond his or her own self. The work targets imposed by the organization would keep pressure on us, creating a sense of urgency. We would try to balance this speed with an inner calm, drawing peace from meditation. And so ultimately, hopefully, we would come to experience a curious yet exhilarating dynamic tension.

For the moment, though, until we received our first postings, we were a bit free. None of us really knew what lay ahead. The others were headed to India soon. Ananta, in fact, had already gone on ahead. Because of my poor health, I would be staying longer in Singapore, to rest. For now, I was what was known as a "floating worker." I was afloat in the world, afloat in organizational channels. And while the others swam vigorously, I floated, contentedly, in the South China Sea.

Singapore. Sparkling isle. Free trade pendant dangling from the necklace of the Malay pensinsula. A lot of money was to be made in this city; its new boulevards were lined with palm trees, its skyscape with towering apartment buildings. And its civil arteries posted with draconian laws: no spitting in public, jail time for grafitti, all under the watchful eyes of the authoritarian Prime Minister Lee Kwan Yew.

I loved the exotic street names: Changi, Jurong, Ang Mo Kio. Sembawang, Orchard, Bukit Timah. Downtown with colonial grace stood the Raffles Hotel, where Joseph Conrad, Somerset Maugham, and Andre Malraux each had lived and written for a time.

If we couldn't yet go to the actual India, we could visit Serangoon Road. Here Sindhi merchants hawked saris, silver necklaces, and *dosa*. Here lived the famous parrot astrologer: a customer whispered his name and birth date into the bird's ear, and the parrot pecked out a card with the right fortune on it. Slight scents of tamarind, jasmine, and turmeric wafted between posters of Hanuman, Krsna, Shiva, and Christ, in veritable deity department stores.

The Singapore jagrti was a large house on Wilkinson Road with a grassy front yard, not far from the ocean. It had a nice meditation hall, a courtyard where we often took our meals, a number of bedrooms, and a homemade aviary in the front yard, with a few tropical birds (though none of them, as far as I knew, had mastered astrology).

Each morning, one of the monks strummed a guitar at 4:45 a.m. I lurched upright, kicked off my blankets, stumbled to the bathroom to splash water on my face, and then with the others padded to the meditation hall. Coming out of a period of intense practice in Davao, I appreciated the sense of continuity. I also appreciated the slight relaxing of training center-pitch discipline. Nevertheless, the room had good vibes, and so I often slipped into concentration.

My memory is tacked with Polaroids of the monks here, like German Dada, who I'd known in Bangkok, still playing his flute.

"You are here?" he said to me, smiling. "I like it very much."

There was also an American monk, an admirer of W. H. Auden. Outside engaged in various work during the day, in the evening he quietly scribbled in his notebook, or, lying on his bedroll, stared off in to the distance. One day to everyone's surprise he announced the imminent publication of a book of short stories and poems.

A dada originally from Hong Kong was the quiet, somewhat awkward jagrti manager. He bought half-rotting fruit to save money, boxes of darkening bananas, mounds of squishy papayas. And the Regional Secretary always yelled at him. "Why do you buy this garbage?"

"But it's much cheaper."

"Yes, I'm sure it is. Nobody can eat it. We have enough money. Don't impose your own karma on everyone else."

The Regional Secretary, a steady Italian, worked in his office all day long. As RS, it was his job to oversee the projects of Singapore and Malaysia: the collection of relief goods to be sent to natural disaster sites in other parts of Asia; several preschools in Malaysia; meditation classes; a small import-export business. He worked long hours; one day he accidentally sliced his thumb with an exacto knife and had to take a few days off.

"I guess," he said, "God wanted me to slow down a little."

Prakash and the RS stood in the kitchen one morning, arguing. I could hear their staccato voices drift through the house as I sat in a front room doing some editing work.

From what I could gather, RS had assigned Prakash to clean the kitchen from top to bottom. For the past few weeks, our brazen Nigerian brother had been incrementally resisting the authority of the RS. Now he crossed a line.

"Do what?" he shouted. "I won't do that!"

"Yes, you will."

"I won't."

"We'll see about that."

RS got on the phone, contacted the Sectorial Secretary, who was in Manila for a meeting, and let him know what was going on.

For not following orders, Prakash was sent back to Davao for retraining. Such a possibility was part of the life of obedience we had embraced. To those of us who had to put up with him in the Singapore jagrti, in some ways it was a relief to see Prakash go. He could be such a headache. And yet, to have just come out of the training center, ready for the world, ready to change the world, and then be sent back…it was a hard thing.

After I found my footing a bit, I set up a booth at a health fair in Bukit Timah, where I sold books and signed people up for yoga classes. One nice young Chinese man, attracted by our philosophy, sat and talked with me for hours. He later came to the jagrti to learn meditation and became active in our relief work.

I also chatted with the twenty year-old son of the fruit seller whose shop we frequented. We talked about spirituality, the importance of doing service. The great saints and religious figures of the world, I told him, got their egos out of the way—they sacrificed for the good of the community. He seemed receptive. One day he drew me aside and told me he had something important to say.

"I need an operation," he began. "I will lead a good life; I will do meditation. Only, will you give me one of your kidneys?"

Stunned, at first I didn't know what to say.

"I...I cannot."

"But you said it is good to sacrifice."

"Yes, but, but this, well, I have a lot of work to do. And my own health is not that great."

He looked down. "But you said..."

Once we commit ourselves to serving others, how do we negotiate the limits of that service? How much are we supposed to give? Examples of service and sacrifice were all around me. Most parents, certainly, put off their own gratification, scraped, saved, went without, so that their kids could have a better life. These days I know someone who *has* donated a kidney to a friend, and I'm in awe of her sacrifice. Maybe, in another lifetime, I would have done the same. But the circumstances in Singapore, and my health situation meant that it just wasn't the right time.

The question swam into tight focus, though. What was the best utilization of my energy, my talents, and my difficult body? How could I best serve?

The incident made me reflect more deeply on one potential meaning of being a monk—letting things come and go in a free flow of resources. And this in turn led to me start thinking about finances. None of us new acharyas really had any money, although we were beginning to feel our way into this gray area. In the training center, of course, we'd had no need of it, bobbing along in embryonic security.

RS impressed on me the importance of a steady source of income. At the moment he had the responsibility to provide food for us, but a few brothers had received donations and could buy small things, a snack in the marketplace, a new pair of slippers. I heard that some trainees in Calcutta whipped up a batch of fresh yogurt straight from the ashram cow each morning and put it up for sale. These forays were a prelude to what lay ahead in the field, the necessity of developing financial stability.

After all, some of us might eventually be overseeing service projects that involved substantial input and outlay of cash.

Some months later, when I was in India, I would encounter the famous fury of Dada PV, a senior monk of the mission. One of my trainee brothers had no money for food, so I approached Dada asking if some could be arranged. He asked how I was getting by, and I remarked that my new in-charge had given me a little money, so I was fine. His bright eyes pierced me for a moment, and then, a sudden fit of pique kindled, he raged, "Then why don't you share what you have with him? What kind of *sannyasi* are you?"

I was struck. He was right, although it also seemed that I couldn't give all my money away. But I'd dedicated my life to serving others. Openness, a sense of surrender, was at the root of our practice. At the same time we had to be practical and learn how to manage our finances. A tension lay between these two poles.

For a few weeks I went to Malaysia and spent time in Ipoh, where four years earlier I'd hung out with the margiis. When I'd last seen them, I'd been new to this part of the world, a shy boy. Now I was more mature. And I was an acharya, with the organization's buoyant support beneath me. They treated me as such and arranged a lecture for me at the Hindu Club.

The members of this club were all South Indians, all men. They met in an open-air pavilion, where pictures of Shiva and Parvatii hung prominently on the one solid wall next to a small shrine with offerings of fresh coconuts and marigold garlands. Cultural influences from the Indian religious tradition existed in AM, but margiis didn't consider themselves Hindus, partly because of AM's strong social revolutionary thrust and opposition to many Hindu practices such as the caste system, or the use of dowry. And some aspects of Hinduism simply seemed dogmatic— the multiple deity worship, the endless ritual. Baba had drawn a distinction between the Vedic tradition, closely tied to Hinduism, and the Tantric, a more practice-based, organic spiritual tradition.

People at the Hindu Club struck me as sincere, but they also seemed fairly set in their ways and not so interested in personal transformation. Still, who knew when and where you might meet someone for whom our ideas resonated?

It was a fasting day. I arrived, dressed in my uniform, as the men were sitting down for their meal.

"Please join us," the organizer said.

"I'm sorry, I'm fasting today."

"Oh, yes? Then just take some fruits, or some tea."

"No, thank you. I fast without food or water."

"Arrre, you are very disciplined," he said, and waggled his head. He was respectful of, if a little puzzled by, my resolve.

I closed my eyes, calmed my mind, and began.

"It is practice, actual spiritual experience, and not belief, which counts on the spiritual path." I quoted from one of Baba's books, a passage about pilgrimage: "There is no need to travel to holy sites, to bathe in so-called holy rivers, rather, it's best to turn inward and meditate." I added some description of the eight limbs of *astaunga* yoga. The men smiled and nodded, some of them lifting their palms in appreciation.

When I finished, the host hastened to the stage. "Let us thank our young American friend, Dadaji, for his enlightening remarks." I received a round of applause.

Some acharyas are powerful public speakers—thunderous orators in the Indian style. Others are thoughtful, well-spoken, and sure of themselves. There are those who say they overcame obstacles in communicating to audiences with the help of some mysterious force. I'd heard stories of workers who barely knew the language in which they spoke, but, upon surrendering, felt a flow of words come. I'd also heard about simple people who impressed a crowd of intellectuals with the clarity of their expression.

I wasn't a great speaker. I had no miraculous experience that day. Yet I also felt that I hadn't given this talk on my own. I'd had some help. If this was learning to surrender, to let go of my ego, I found it as pleasant as floating on the blue waves of the Johor Straits.

"You've received damaged goods," the Danish dada joked. Recently posted to Singapore, he'd been struck down by hepatitis as soon as he arrived. Knocked flat for a month, he asked me to go to the market and buy plastic bags full of sugarcane juice for him. I did, watching the revolving hand-press rollers mash the bamboo sticks of cane, sweet green froth pouring out the other end.

"Sugarcane juice contains glucose," the Dane explained. "The doctor wants me to drink more glucose. A cure for hepatitis. Don't worry," he continued, "Doctor also says hepatitis is only passed through intimate contact. So wash all my plates and spoons, and everyone should be fine."

How, then, did I contract it? Did it lurk, ready to pounce on new victims, in household objects? In the kitchen? In the bathroom?

Feeling ill at ease one day, I asked a friend to give me a foot rub. I loved his intense massages. Pressing his thumb deeply into the fleshy ball of my foot, he explained that each part of the foot was linked through the nerves to a specific point in the body. By massaging the foot one is stimulating and benefiting the corresponding organs.

"Here are the lungs," he said, pressing firmly. "Here, the intestines."

"And here," he said, digging in, "is the liver."

"Yeowwww!"

I bolted upright, the lingering sense of unease suddenly crystallizing into a deeper pain and nausea. In the next few days the metamorphosing color of my skin confirmed my fears. This time it was not my foot, but my liver swelling up, as my body drained itself of energy. Suddenly I was a yellow man, the bile from my gall bladder migrating to just below the surface of my skin, and the irises of my eyes, too, chameleon-like, shifting from hazel to gold. In the mirror I looked like some magical creature.

A hospital visit pronounced it Non-A Non-B hepatitis. *What did this mean?* One doctor at first claimed it to be Hep B, but this turned out to be a false positive. Another doctor hypothesized that it was simply an inflammation of the liver, a kind of hepatitis, but not Hepatitis with a capital "H." Confusion reigned, and I would never be clear about the exact cause of so much pain.

Once again I was flat on my back for weeks, my abdomen taut and sore. My body felt like a war zone. I did my meditation lying down, and spent my time watching videos and listening to the parakeets chatter from the front yard. After some time, I dragged myself out to the front porch to sit in the sun. From there I could watch old men across the street twisting and swooping as they practiced Tai Chi.

If I had to wait to go to India because of poor health when I first came out of the training center, the hepatitis pushed my departure back even further. I would have to rest, recuperate, and this would take time. I would stay in Singapore for months, much longer than Valmiki, who went on ahead for his final exam in India, and then to his posting in Argentina, before I even reached India. Even Prakash would be back through Singapore before I left, his retraining completed, seemingly more willing to follow orders.

There are, it seems, energies in our bodies that can be coaxed and regulated, through eating the right food, performing the right exercises, even thinking the right thoughts. But there are also blind forces over which we have no control—live wires skittering back and forth across the pavement of our viscera, chain-reaction meltdowns radiating fallout over the grazing lands of our cells.

I knew that through my spiritual practices my psyche had begun to be transformed, knots loosening, emotional problems I'd faced since adolescence dwindling in significance. But now, it was as if the arena of struggle was shifting. Now my body was assuming the role of a stumbling block.

On a level beyond my control, something had waited for me, floating, something which would have a great impact on my long-term health, a reckoning of accounts for which my immune system would claim insufficient funds. I'd hoped, as a new acharya, to come out of the gates running, to make my mark, to please my guru. I would go on to India for the final acharya exam, and then to my posting in South Korea. I would throw myself into the work and accomplish many things, but always with the companionship of pain, fatigue, and a body that couldn't quite do everything I wanted it to do.

Perhaps the lesson to be learned was the inevitability of human frailty, of physical breakdown. If so, it was a hard lesson.

For now, I floated.

Chapter Twenty-Eight

After a year of working and resting in Singapore, my health improved to the point that I was able to go to India for final exams with Baba.

As I flew into Calcutta, I was mindful of the Indian government's standing threat to deport foreign margiis, the resentment and suspicion the government had for Baba and his organization. I recalled the care I and other margiis had had to take while traveling to Ananda Nagar and other parts of India. So I was cautious, on the off chance I was searched or detained in the airport, not to have carried any incriminating evidence: no AM literature, no addresses in my datebook, and certainly not my uniform.

Standing in Dum Dum Airport's immigration line, I even pretended to smoke a cigarette. It was one way to throw officials off the trail, since margiis stood out in an airport crowd. The men often had beards, wore their hair long, and there was something else about them, a spark, perhaps, in their eyes. But, as everyone knew, they didn't smoke. For the last four years I'd been working hard to shed aspects of my past, but in this moment I needed to assume a few of the stereotypical qualities of the ugly American.

"I'm a tourist," I told the man at the immigration counter; it was the least controversial purpose. And it worked. I made it through. I also fed the taxi driver a red herring by first having him take me downtown, switching taxis, and then heading to the jagrti, just to be on the safe side. I'd heard that immigration spies sometimes followed travelers from the airport to see if they ended up at AM jagrtis.

So I'd been careful. But one day during my stay at Tiljala I had an experience that gave me pause. Every day I took a rickshaw from the small village near our ashram—VIP Nagar—to Balleygunge where I could catch a bus to Baba's house. And returned home retracing my route. One day on the road separating VIP Nagar from a small market at the edge of the city ward, a strange man stood and stared at me. He had a conspiratorial air about him as he drank in my appearance. He was still there when I returned. Why would anyone stand there so long on the highway, so close to our buildings?

I soon forgot about it, though, as I was having final acharya exams with Baba. During these exams Baba requested all of us new acharyas to "hold high the banner of universalism." He also encouraged me to read French literature, a suggestion I can only hypothesize had to do with that tradition's history of depicting social problems. He quizzed us briefly on questions of philosophy and asked us to demonstrate certain asanas. It was a wonderful experience, the culmination of our time in the training center, and a gift before we headed off to our postings.

After a few weeks, it was time to fly out again from Dum Dum. I had been given my first official posting, assigned to work in East Asia, specifically South Korea, and I was flying to Bangkok where I would apply for a Korean visa. Being validated by Baba as an acharya was such a wonderful experience that I was probably a little distracted as I prepared to leave the country. Usually cautious about what I packed, this time I grew a little careless, perhaps even cocky: I had two newly published PROUT books tucked deep inside one of my bags.

Arriving at the terminal, I sat in the waiting room for a while and tried to figure the best strategy for getting in line. Board too early and immigration had plenty of time to interrogate you. Rushing through at the last minute sometimes worked, although this had also been known to arouse suspicion. I flipped idly through a magazine, singing kiirtan quietly to myself.

Finally I got in line and made it to the counter, and as the man paged through my passport, I watched a uniformed intelligence officer, very intelligent-*looking*, approach from a small room behind the desk, whisper something to another officer, and then motion for me to step out of line. The other passengers perked up, intrigued. I was escorted to a room where the man asked me to be seated. I sank back in a hard plastic chair. A huge map of India covered one wall.

"What brings you to India?" He was a cool customer.

"Pleasure, mostly. I'm here as a tourist." My heart was pounding, but I could be cool, too.

"Where did you visit?"

"Oh, Delhi, Agra, Benaras. You have some beautiful places here."

"Thank you. You have praised our country. Where did you stay in Calcutta?"

"Oh, the Hotel Raj." It was a well-known tourist hotel, fairly nice. "Say, what's this all about anyway?"

The man looked down at my feet. I was wearing cheap Indian rubber thongs. "Why aren't you wearing shoes?" he asked suspiciously.

"Oh, that. Well, at the hotel I put my shoes outside my door to be cleaned, and someone stole them. I didn't have time to get new ones." He frowned.

"You can call the hotel," I pitched in. "They'll vouch for me."

"Do you know Ananda Marga?"

I cleared my throat. There it was. "No, who's that? Some politician?"

"What about Baba?"

"Baba? Listen, I'd better not miss my plane. What's going on here?"

"May we search your bags?"

What could I say? "Suit yourself." I walked over to the airline counter and identified my bags, which had not yet been sent to the plane. Another man joined the first, and they opened my suitcase and began pulling items from it, until they came to an orange T-shirt. "Why do you have a T-shirt this color?"

I almost laughed. It seemed a stretch for them to link T-shirts to anything. "What do you mean? What's special about this color?" The men looked at each other. Then, in a compartment zippered away and wrapped in a shawl, they withdrew a small book—*New Aspects of PROUT.* The first man smiled.

"What's this?"

"I bought it at a bookstore downtown. It looked interesting."

"Of course you did. We'll keep this."

The Thai Airlines officials were getting antsy, inquiring about the delay. The plane, apparently, was being held for me. How was this going to play out? It hadn't yet struck me that I was about to be banned from ever entering India again, that I was falling victim to an unfair policy tied to events years in the past that had nothing to do with me. And that this would, in future, cause me lots of difficulty.

Given the go-ahead by the intelligence official, I hurried toward the boarding gate.

"It's OK," the man said to one of the Thai Airlines staff, while scribbling in a notebook. "He can go now."

I showed my boarding pass to the frowning airlines attendant.

"But," the officer added loudly, "he won't be back."

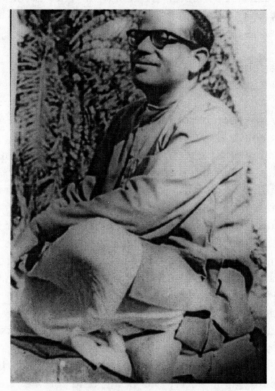

Prabhat Ranjan Sarkar (1921-1990)
Also known as Shrii Shrii Anandamurti and Baba
by the followers of Ananda Marga

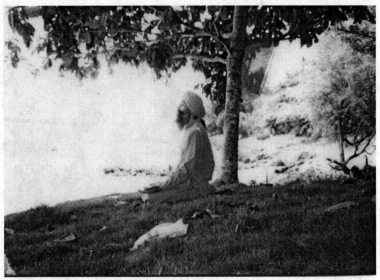

Dada Cidanada, in charge of Davao Acharya Training Center
in the Philippines c. 1986

A group of monks-in-training near Davao, Philippines

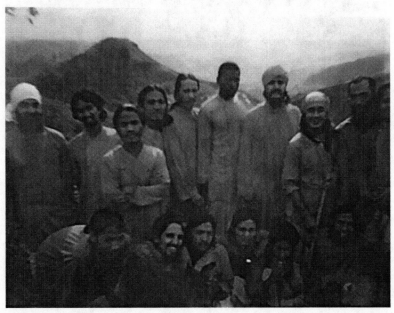

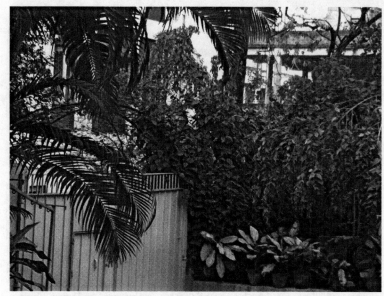

Gate outside Anandamurti's house in Lake Gardens, Calcutta
where Baba would sit and listen to people singing Prabhat Samgiit

The author meditating in Korean forest c. 1989

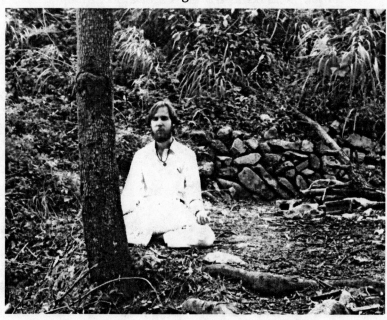

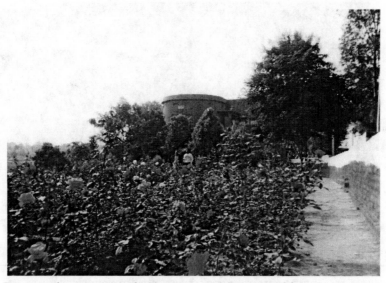

Rose gardens at Ananda Nagar, an AM sustainable community in West Bengal, India

Author with several Korean margiis in the hills above Seoul, Korea c. 1989

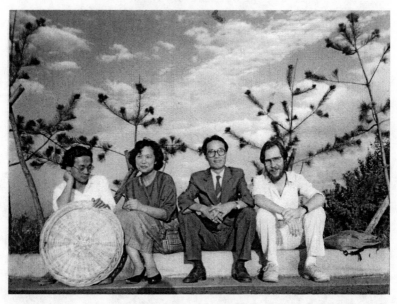

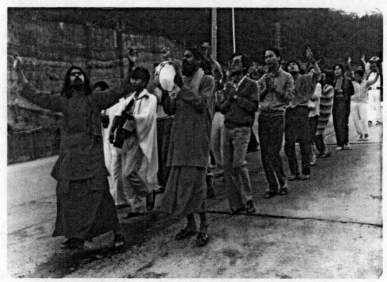

Singing kirtan in the streets of a Taiwanese city,
led by Dada IK (left) who worked with the author
while in Japan c. mid-1980's

Author (back center) with Nepalese margii family, after having
crossed the border from India c. 1990

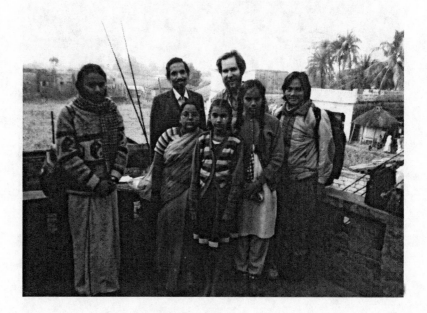

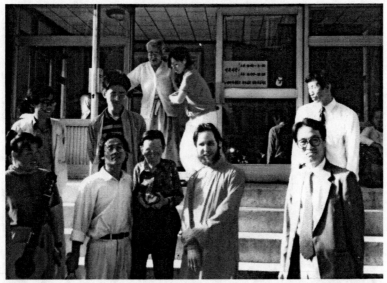

Doing social service at an old folks' home in Seoul, Korea c. 1989

Author (center seated) with college students following a talk
at a university in Pusan, Korea

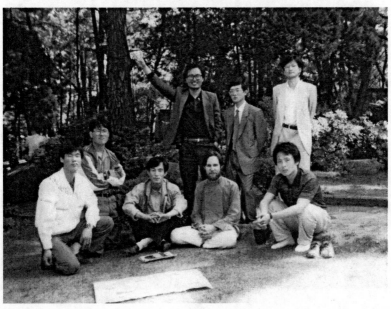

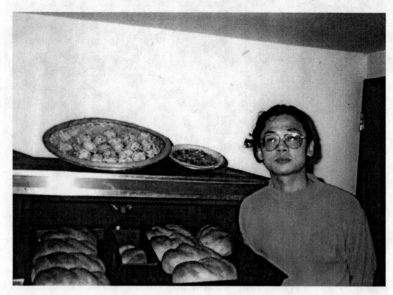

Jiitendra, Korean margii, baking bread in the AM bakery in Seoul

Land outside Jeonju, Korea, purchased to develop an AM center

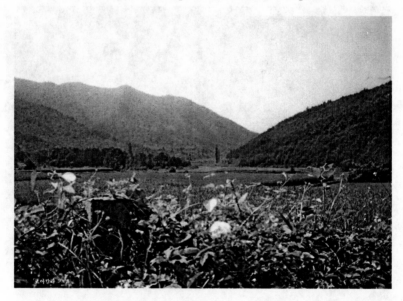

Part Four — Seoul

CHAPTER TWENTY-NINE

My plane touched down at Kimpo Airport in January of 1989. The city of Seoul was surrounded on three sides by towering, rugged mountain ranges, offshoots of which split the city like swollen knuckles running across a giant fist. Many of the city's buildings were built into the shadows of these craggy cliffs. It was cold, but sunny. Armed military guards stood on alert throughout the terminal, staring straight ahead into an unfathomable middle distance, their helmets glinting in the sun, a reminder that the country was still, technically, at war with its cousin, North Korea.

I'd spent the last two weeks shadowing my new boss, Dada S, the Sectorial Secretary for East Asia, around Taiwan. I was getting a feel for how the organization operated there, before taking up my duties as the new Regional Secretary for Seoul. Dada S was no doubt waiting to see what kind of worker he'd gotten for the sector. Earlier I'd mentioned that I'd studied English Literature, which seemed to please him. "Ah, a literary man!" he said. "You'll be able to give good talks, then." That remained to be seen.

Taiwan was the yardstick for measuring success for AM in East Asia. Things were going gangbusters with schools, yoga classes, a booming bakery business, hundreds of dedicated margiis, and some recently acquired land for a sustainable community. Drawing on a long Chinese tradition of meditative practice, but one uninterrupted by Communist suppression, the people here seemed inclined toward a subtle spirituality. They were also incredible cooks, and we'd enjoyed their hospitality all across the island.

Over lunch one day I'd chatted with another monk who'd been in East Asia for years. "Going to Seoul?" he asked. "Hmmm. You'll do fine. Still, it's a hard field. Not many margiis. Some acharyas have left the mission from there..."

This did not worry me. I would never leave.

I knew little about Korea, knew no one there, and didn't speak the language. But there would be time to learn, as I anticipated being here for many years. I would be one of five or six acharyas scattered across the country. And as ephemeral as such a thing may sometimes seem, I felt a measure of what I interpreted as grace—a warm fullness in my chest, a sense of peace and clarity. I had high hopes, though my health was ragged. But I kept in mind something Baba had said about making the fullest utilization of strength you have. Once you've done that, extra strength to complete the task will come.

Exiting the arrivals gate in Seoul, I noticed a young woman and a middle-aged man scanning the crowd. They spotted me and though I was not in uniform, something clicked in their eyes. This bearded, gentle-looking Westerner must be the new RS. I also noticed that the man looked surprised—at my age? My frail body? Perhaps he was expecting someone more seasoned.

Slightly awkward introductions all around.

"Are you Dada?"

"Yes, I am."

"Namaskar, so nice to meet you."

"Nice to meet you."

This was Liilavati, earnest art student, and Dhruva, an older man who owned a small engineering firm in Daegu. Dhruva picked up my bag, and they ushered me to the train for the ride into the city. Out the window, farmhouses and green fields gave way to ever-denser neighborhoods, until the train slipped underground. A man with a coarse face and wiry hair walked the length of our car, laying a pack of gum in the lap of each passenger. Then he stood at the head of the car and made his appeal in a lackluster cadence.

"Selling something," Liilavati explained to me.

Come to think of it, so was I.

Seoul bustled and seethed. Student demonstrations or "demos" against the military dictatorship were exploding in the streets, as were the government's retaliatory measures. At each subway stop plainclothes goons whispered into handheld radios and stopped pedestrians, especially college students, in order to search their bags. Squadrons of riot police lounged beside armored buses in the streets, waiting for the command to mobilize. I was, it appeared, now living in a police state. Yet I was excited and intrigued by it all. I was eager to observe resistance to oppression on the ground.

The jagrti was a two-bedroom apartment in Seokyo-dong, at the nexus of four major universities, smack in the middle of the sea of student unrest. But there were oases of quiet. With their sweepingly curved red tile roofs the houses in our neighborhood looked vaguely Chinese, and ancient. Outside of the narrow cobblestone alley leading to our house, a sweet potato vendor rotated his big metal drum of an oven. The smell was irresistible; we bought a few for lunch.

A retreat had been scheduled for that very weekend, so after a bite to eat and a brief nap, we set out again by train, heading for the mountains south of Daegu. This would be typical of the pace I assumed as the new RS, arriving in a new place one day, then heading to a meeting halfway across the country the next morning. For a time, I was able to keep it up.

Our train sped down the peninsula from the northern mountains into the great southern plain. A sparkling river danced alongside the tracks and then disappeared into a mountain pass; this country was gorgeous. From Daegu we took a local bus to the end of the line, and got down next to a dilapidated *makkali* shop with its strong smell of rice wine. We were headed for a small country house in the mountains, the property of one of Dhruva's friends in a place called Chisan-dong. My head was full of plans.

This was it, cast into a leadership role at last. I was nervous, but the half-hour walk up the hill to the retreat site gave me courage. The landscape here was the most beautiful I'd seen in five years of travels— towering pines mirrored in pristine lakes, fold after fold of the mountain appearing above us like a paper fan. I'd never been to Switzerland, but surely this was what the lower Alps looked like. We came within sight of the house, and there for the first time I met many of the Korean margiis, the thirty or so college students and middle-aged family people attending the retreat. They welcomed me warmly, and then we all sat down to do that thing we do, that thing that had brought us all together.

After meditation, a feast: freshly picked mountain greens with sesame; carrots fried in honey and chili; sweet black beans and lettuce; tofu marinated in a sauce of *shoyu;* sesame oil, chili paste and sugar; pickled cucumber and cabbage kimchi; hot rice and seaweed, washed down with sparkling spring water toted down from the mountain.

Sitting at the heated table, we sang kiirtan for a while, our eyes closed in appreciation. Then I followed the others' lead as they wrapped crisp lettuce leaves around white rice and barley, added spiced bean paste, and popped the concoctions into their mouths. These people knew how to enjoy food!

After dinner everyone threw on jackets and we walked the country road, past a little evangelical Christian church down the way. A hymn even now was floating across the vale, a tune I remembered from childhood, though again, the words were unknown to me. The night was clear and cold, strange constellations of stars smeared across the firmament, incredibly bright and close here on the mountain. Returning to the house, we wrapped ourselves in blankets. Someone brought out sweet pears, the kind I had enjoyed in Japan, and we competed, laughing, to see who could carve the longest, most unbroken peel.

We spent much of the night singing some spiritual songs, but also Korean folk songs like *Arirang*. Everyone was expected to sing, especially this newcomer. So, of course, I chose a Prabhat Samgiit song.

Who are you just arrived, unknown traveler? Who are you who came into my heart?

Watching these people sway and hug one another, I began to pick up on a subtle difference in the way people related to each other here. One word in particular I heard over and over: "Uri," "Our" or "we." Koreans, it seemed, always referred to "our house," never "my house," and to "our country," not "my country." The incessant "I – I – I" of the West was out of place here. Rhythms of one spirit flowed between these several hearts. At first I felt myself more keenly an individual, but after some time I began to feel pulled into the almost embryonic sense of connectedness. I would probably never be able to participate fully in this—in fact that was not my goal—but I liked the feeling.

We slept, the men and women in separate buildings, wrapped in thick patterned blankets on the linoleum floor, above the burning *undol*, a dug-out hearth underneath the building. A fire kept stoked in this pit beneath the house radiated cozy heat up through the floor. Every few hours one of the brothers ventured outside to add more branches. It was a toasty heating method, but difficult to control—once you added too much fuel, there was no way to turn down the heat, and at some point the room became unbearably warm.

I was happy, excited to feel that I might really fit in here, and slept deeply. During the night I rolled off my blanket, but did not wake up, and in the morning saw that my bare calf had been seared by the overheated floor. I had received a burn from the *undol*, a mark I carry to this day.

It was my body's initiation into the intensity of the relationships here, and into the mysteries of this culture which I would grow to love, and its claim on me.

A couple of student activists attending the retreat were interested in learning more about PROUT. Over breakfast one of them filled me in a little on the student movement, telling me how they were pushing for reunification and an overthrow of military rule. Student radicals had a tremendous track record in Korea. Most of the major social changes over the past 40 years had been prodded by their activism. Good, I thought, these are the types of dynamic people we need to attract.

But Dhruva, old enough to remember the war with the Communists, was suspicious. "Do not trust them," he told me. Sometimes charming, Dhruva could also be stubborn and childlike, and once he felt slighted, I learned, he bore a grudge. This was only one of many conflicts playing out among the margiis. Most of these tensions were, in these early days, occurring beneath my radar.

After breakfast we sat for a meeting. My idea was to encourage each of the margiis to get involved with some sort of project. I whipped out my list of project ideas and asked one sister to translate for me.

"Umm, thank you for your warm welcome. I'd like to discuss a few possible activities. Ultimately it is up to you what we do—I hope you'll get involved." With hearty bravado, down the list I went: A service project. Teaching yoga classes. Organizing philosophy classes. Starting a cooperative business. Purchasing land for a retreat center. Expanding publications.

Although AM had maintained a presence in Korea for ten years, few of these more concrete goals had been established. Perhaps this was due to the oppressive atmosphere of military rule. There was the language gap, too, between acharyas posted here and margiis. Or perhaps it was because Koreans were fiercely independent, and distrusted outsiders.

As the meeting went on, I noticed Dhruva had been frowning for some time. Now he began to speak forcefully in Korean. From what I could gather, the margiis had been trying to develop a publications policy, but were in disagreement over the details. The argument escalated, the meeting threatening to deteriorate. I called for a ten-minute break and stepped outside for some fresh air. This was not what I'd expected. I didn't know these people and it wasn't my place to mediate between them, not on my first weekend here.

But it was, in the end, a successful retreat. Thanks to lots of kiirtan, meditation, stories, and good food, people seemed inspired. Exhausted after it was over, I stayed on at Chi-san for a few days to relax. Several brothers remained with me. I felt a strong connection with one of them—Om Karnath (OK), a young student of German philosophy who spoke very good English.

At breakfast OK scraped out the rice stuck to the bottom of the pot. "My mother used to feed me this," he said. "You see, you soak the burnt rice in water and drink the soup. Koreans mostly ate this after the war; so now when we eat it, it's a kind of, what do you say, collective memory of that era's poverty."

OK's intelligence was matched by sharp wit and a deadpan delivery, and he had us rolling on the floor with his stories.

"Five people," he began, "were meditating in a row at a retreat last year. Harideva, you know him? The president of AM in Korea. He is sixty years old. He began to doze. He nodded forward, nodded to the side, then he jerked up. Finally, he fell over backwards, and made this noise, 'Ohh!' in surprise."

"With my eyes closed, you see, I thought Harideva was making the noise of someone deep in concentration; you know, he was slipping into *samadhi*. So I got inspired, and resolved to concentrate more deeply," OK smiled, "while poor Harideva was lying on the floor, rubbing his head!"

Also staying in an adjacent cabin at the mountain house was an old no-nonsense Buddhist monk, a friend of Dhruva's. I watched him stroll purposefully up the hill in his brown robes, stopping to pluck greens from along the roadside for cooking, or to pick up a piece of trash and place it in a plastic bag. When he heard my health was poor, he was quick to suggest some native herbs.

Late into the night we heard him clacking the resonant wooden block designed to help focus the mind for "Son" meditation, Korea's version of Zen. Then he sang a traditional Buddhist song, his voice all guttural yodel, which the others translated for me— "I am a monk, I am married to the mountain. She is my wife, I have no other."

Good song.

I admired his straightforward approach to the monk's life. He seemed to embody a quote I discovered by Korean Buddhist Chinul: "Adept people in everything are like empty boats riding the waves, buoyantly going along with nature."

I could imagine living here for a time on the mountain, surrounded by the woods, observing the seasons, meditating into them, picking herbs from the roadside, being part of a small community, or living alone, working and eating and growing older. Those few days on Chi-san were a wonderful introduction to Korean life for me, particularly a kind of traditional, now-disappearing rural ethos. Long after I returned to Seoul, I recalled it with pleasure, remembering Chinul's words.

But I was also eager to get back to Seoul and plunge into the plans and projects I had in mind. Pressure from the organization to *establish* AM in Korea weighed on me. But I was invested, too. I wanted to do something good. On the late bus from Daegu to the capital, winding down the mountainside, the lights of the city sparkled like a great celestial realm, welcoming me to my new home.

I keep a photograph from that time (p. 175): Four people sitting on a curb, high in the hills of southern Seoul, the descending terraces of a valley dropping off behind them, as if they're perched on the edge of the world. Because of the angle of the photo, and the drop-off, the background appears like a stage scrim, rolled out across the middle distance. Four tree saplings rise, one behind each of the four friends, their conifer branches dissecting the blue sky. Beautiful white clouds scud across this gorgeous sky. The four had just come from spending time with old folks at a retirement home up in the hills, one of our regular service projects. Three of these people are Korean, and one is a Westerner.

On the left sits Jiitendra, a young man in his 20's with gentle features, holding a large circular wicker bakery tray in front of him, which covers the bottom half of his body. His long hair is pinned in a ponytail, he props his face on his elbow, and with a faint half-smile, he looks down and off to the right. Son of a conservative Christian preacher, at an early age he rebelled, became an artist, and went off to do his own thing, part of which included moving into the yoga and meditation center I oversaw. Uninhibited, he existed in another world. I heard he once danced naked in the street outside his art college. Demonstrating a bemused distance from the organization's hierarchies and rules, he turned out to be a good counterbalance for me, as he was always testing me, slightly mocking any tendency I had to take my organizational role too seriously.

Next to him in the photo, a woman in her late twenties, conservatively dressed, with ankle length dress and sensible shoes, tilts slightly toward Jiitendra, but is looking away from the camera in the other direction from him. She also smiles slightly, as if her high expectations have been met, as if the circumstances of the day have coalesced around her no-nonsense values. She is here, I believe, because she loves the sense of community, and the yoga exercises, or asanas. Attending regular yoga classes at our Seoul center, she has slowly come to identify herself as part of this group.

Then, in a brown single-breasted suit and tie, feet planted firmly, legs slightly askew, his wide-frame glasses framing 60-year old features is Harideva, the same person who fell over in OK's story. He beams with satisfaction into the camera. We've done something good, his expression says. I have done something good. And though his home life is complicated, and his work drains him, the fact of his commitment to this little yoga group, and the fact that he has assumed a role of leadership satisfies and sustains him through his difficulties. I like him quite a bit.

Then there's me, American monk in his mid-20s, lately arrived in Korea. Not today wearing his monk's orange, but instead clad casually in cream-colored slacks, light short sleeve shirt and tennis shoes. A full beard and longish hair. I'm smiling, too, straight into the camera.

Now 27, and assuming my duties in Seoul, I had begun connecting with people as a leader and as a friend, sometimes having to deal with sensitive egos, investing in the hard slog of building a movement. I was, it's true, no born organizer. I had ideals, but I was a little too quiet to galvanize people. I had gained some measure of selflessness, I guess. Mostly I just wanted to please my guru.

Four people smile out from this photo, wildly different from but comfortable with each other, brought together for the purpose of doing good, each in their own way happy with the day. The camera freezes these four, framed by Korea's green foothills and broad cobalt sky, as they gaze with introspection or distraction or satisfaction into their futures.

And so I settled into the Seoul jagrti, creating a daily routine with the three Koreans who lived there—a university student studying Spanish, Jiitendra, the uninhibited art student, and a military reservist. These brothers and I rose at 5 each day, meditated for an hour or more, did our asanas, and then had a lazy, conversation-filled breakfast, usually rice and *chajang*, a kind of bean soup. We then went about the day's business.

That first Sunday, I remember, there was a good turnout for group meditation, 15 or so people, including a young woman who wheeled herself up to our front door in a wheelchair. We carried her up the stairs and arranged a seat for her inside. "The kiirtan music flowing over me was a healing experience," she told me later. What could be a better validation of the work we were trying to do?

Liilavati, perhaps the most active of the margiis and someone who would go on to become an acharya herself, soon arranged for me to lead a seminar at a college outside of Seoul. It took an hour by bus to get there. In the lecture room, she translated as I talked about the benefits of meditation to a roomful of students. "You may find you will be better able to concentrate," I advised them, "and do better in your studies."

Twelve young men agreed to learn, a regular assembly line. As I instructed them individually after the lecture, Liilavati translated my instructions. It remained to be seen whether any would take it seriously. Teaching meditation via translation was not the right way to go about it. There was too much room for misunderstanding in getting across what was at heart a subjective practice, but what else could I do until I learned the language?

During that first month Harideva's father died, and Liilavati encouraged me to attend the wake. We took the subway across town and from the station walked a few blocks to the modest one-story home with a small stone fence. A huge garlanded photo of Harideva's elderly father stared from the vestibule of the house. Visitors milled, eating and drinking. Harideva stood at the door in a brown suit. "Thank you for coming," he kept repeating. "Thank you for coming." From the look on his face I could tell that he appreciated his spiritual family being there.

Here I met a number of other margiis, including Kapildeva, a retired Army general well into his 70s, still wearing a crew cut, still cultivating an intimidating presence. Ten years earlier he'd faced serious illness, and like many Koreans of his generation had turned to natural healing methods, including asanas and vegetarianism. The regimen cured him, and after that he brought his full military enthusiasm to an advocacy of yoga. Though bowed by time, he maintained an air of army decorum and officer's gravitas. He liked to bark orders at the younger margiis, who felt uncomfortable around him.

Respect for elders, filial piety, an ongoing relationship with the ancestors, all the traditional aspects of Korean culture were on display at this wake, but also evident in the older margiis' behavior. It was behavior stemming from Confucian times when society had been strictly structured along lines of familial and governmental authority.

"They send the most inexperienced acharyas here to Korea, right?" one of these older margiis asked me brusquely. How to respond to this? It was true that Korea seemed low on the totem pole of East Asia, organizationally speaking. Most workers went to Taiwan where the margiis were many and devoted, or to Japan, where you could raise money. Young acharyas like myself were often sent first to Seoul, as if to be tested, to see whether we could make it here.

I *was* a relatively young man, thrust into a society where age was the critical factor for determining the nature of any relationship. The younger margiis addressed me as "Dada Ge-sa," suffixing my name with a sign of respect. But it would take time to understand how to navigate relationships with the older people. They were from another era, a time in which male elders ruled, and women and young people knew their place. I listened respectfully to Kapildeva and Dhruva and the other older men, but often felt that a new approach was needed in developing the organization here, and sometimes our relationships became strained.

I was an acharya, literally "one who teaches by example," and yet I was not unaware of a certain irony in this. What was my example grounded in? Not years of experience, but the zeal of a young monk. I'd had training, I'd spent time with Baba, I was a hard worker, and I had the resources of the organization behind me. But I also knew that I was young. Earning the respect of all the margiis, becoming a seasoned worker, would take time. So I just plowed ahead, doing what needed to be done, taking baby steps, trying to deal tactfully with whatever came in my path.

Speaking of baby steps. A margii couple—a Korean woman and a Frenchman who taught his mother tongue at a Seoul language academy—had recently had a baby. When the child turned six months they planned to bring him to the jagrti for a celebration, and to receive a spiritual name. I would be doing the naming.

On the appointed day they arrived with the little boy. All the Seoul margiis gathered in the meditation hall in a festive mood, and we began by singing a Prabhat Samgiit song written for this kind of occasion:

Nanir putul tutul tutul. Hath par nache hese hese.

Our little child is just like a doll, wiggling his fingers and toes and smiling…The luster of the celestial world is glowing in his eyes. I will nurture him well.

Each person poured a small cup of water into the little bassinet in which the baby sat, symbolizing a collective commitment to the child's wellbeing. We then all chanted the appropriate mantras.

Oh gracious Brahma, may we be able to provide adequate education for the mental development of this child. The mother and father joined in on another round of pouring water. *May we succeed in effecting the spiritual elevation of this infant.* The tyke gurgled and cooed, splashing his hands in the water, enjoying all the attention.

Then I placed my hand on the child's head, a feeling of affection welling in me. "His name will be Arjuna," I said. "Arjuna was a great spiritual person, a friend of Krsna's." The parents beamed at each other.

The boy looked up at me wonderingly. Tears filled the eyes of many of the margiis.

The ceremony over, everyone congratulated the parents and took turns cradling the baby. We adjourned to the dining room, and enjoyed the potluck feast that had been prepared. I bounced the boy on my knee for a while. Afterwards, as was so common when Koreans gathered, we sang. It was a wonderful afternoon.

And long after the ceremony ended, and these good people had gone home, and I and the other brothers did the washing up, the meaning of the closing mantras lingered in my mind:

May the wind bring blessings with it. May the ocean yield felicity. May our herbs be blissful. May the day and night be sweet.

CHAPTER THIRTY

One day three months after I arrived in Seoul, a brother from Pusan came for a visit. As we prepared a simple dinner, he pointed out that whenever he visited Seoul, the jagrti refrigerator always seemed to be empty.

"You need to keep it full, Dada," he said chirpily, "so that the margiis feel welcome!" I said nothing, as he thought he was doing me a favor. He couldn't realize how much I was struggling simply to pay the rent.

When I'd been in Taipei, Dada S had breezed through an overview of the Seoul financial picture, providing me with a list of people whose regular donations he assured me would cover all expenses. "So there shouldn't be any problem," he'd smiled. "OK?"

Intent on visiting some of the people on Dada's list, I headed for the train station one afternoon, past the cafes with their unintentionally hilarious English names: *Pizza Topic, Falling in Coffee.* I sat on the train for more than an hour, flung around the farthest orbit of Seoul. Alighting from the train, I found the right towering apartment building, went up, met the brother, and together with his wife and baby, enjoyed a nice dinner in his tiny apartment. It turns out that he was more of a sympathizer than an active margii. The evening wore on, but no mention was made of money. I was aware of the need for tact. Finally, when it was time to go, I asked, "Can you…can you help me a little bit?"

He stopped, puzzled, then replied, "Sure, Dada," and went into the other room, bringing out a 10,000 won note (about $12). "Thank you for coming."

Clearly, he was neither accustomed or in a position to support AM on a regular basis. And this turned out to be more common among the people on the list than I'd hoped. The rosy portrait painted by the dada quickly faded. Few people were ready to commit to a monthly donation. And expenses were high: a jagrti in downtown Seoul, travel to the south every weekend, and pressure from Dada S himself to open a place in Daegu. The brothers who lived in the Seoul jagrti helped with rent, and a few other margiis gave donations, but we never seemed to quite meet our expenses. Those who were serious about supporting were often students with little money to spare. The work of building a strong foundation here was yet to be done.

In the meantime I stumbled across one way to make some money: proofing Korean-to-English translations for a local translation company. This business was presided over by a unique figure. From his cluttered office, his desk obscured under teetering piles of manuscripts and books, Mr. Park watched as underlings scurried in and out, dropping off sheaves of paper. "You call this English?" he called after them. "I could tie a pen to my dog's tail and come up with a better translation!"

Though I got a kick out of Mr. Park's antics, the work was drudgery; most of the papers were very technical, dealing, for example, with specs for an undersea telecom cable. A few were interesting. I checked the speech of an automotive company president who hoped to inspire foreign investors with his plans to "invade" and "penetrate" the Chinese market. He wanted to follow the lead of the "advanced countries" by cutting wages and production costs, moving his plants to third world countries where labor was cheaper.

Here spelled out in black and white were the worst inclinations of capitalist business, and I was getting paid to make sure they were expressed in proper English. My Proutist sensibility bristled. I didn't like editing these words, but it was a dissonance I was willing to allow, if it meant I could pay the rent.

Then I remembered something. My predecessor as RS had run a bakery business here. A jolly Swiss, he had been successful in Seoul on many levels. By restarting the bakery I thought I might duplicate that success. Two industrial-sized ovens, the kind you'd see in a pizza restaurant, about three feet across, with two levels of racks, were stored in a spare room at the jagrti. After some discussion, Jiitendra—who tutored art students but needed some extra income—agreed to take on the work, and so one afternoon we dusted off the ovens and fired up the gas.

Jiitendra also accompanied me to a hard-to-find back alley market, where we bought cookie punches, trays, tongs, plastic bags and twisties, and lots of butter, and ordered huge sacks of flour to be delivered by truck to our house.

He and I set about learning to bake, poring over the stained loose-leaf binder of recipes the Swiss had left behind. Several times a week, spreading papers on the floor to catch the mess, we inserted a kiirtan tape into the cassette player, tied on aprons and got down to business. We mixed mountains of barley and whole wheat flour, salt, sugar, and water into the huge stainless steel bowls, kneading, kneading, punching down the dough endlessly, a halo of flour floating in the air around us. Then we loaded the full bread pans into the oven, turned on the gas, and waited.

Finally we unloaded something beautiful. Nothing, it seemed to me, was more satisfying than the sight of those long soft amber-colored loaves, hot and fresh from the oven: the rare pleasure of an end product. Dada BV in Tokyo had sometimes remarked on how difficult it was to gauge one's progress in the spiritual life. It wasn't like mowing the lawn, he said, where you could look back and see, row by row, what you had done. He sometimes longed for more tangible tasks. I could relate. With the bakery at least I had something I could sink my teeth into, a project that required a lot of effort, but seemed to bring people together. And which helped bring in some cash. Every other weekend, I loaded a bag with freshly baked bread and cookies and the occasional pizza and strapped it to my luggage dolly. Then I'd catch a bus either to Jeonju or Daegu, or Pusan, depending on my schedule.

I sold the baked goods to margiis, and later to small neighborhood shops. They were impressed with the rich recipes. And with the increased income, after I'd been in Korea for eight months, we were able to open a jagrti in Daegu. Some of the older margiis felt there was no need for such a center and declined to support it financially. Dhruva, for example, had been close friends with my predecessor, the Swiss, and seemed to feel that no one could measure up to him. I had a sneaking suspicion that he resented my efforts. He gave no money.

But a small cadre of dedicated students, led by Om Karnath, the philosophy student, went to bat for the jagrti, somehow scraping together enough money each month, along with income from the bakery sales, to pay the rent. It was a constant struggle, but it fired a sense of closeness between us. We were in it together, and every month that we made another payment was a shared victory.

After meditation on Sundays, when most of the other margiis had returned home, those students and I pulled on our jackets, laced up our shoes, and went out to stroll the evening streets of Daegu. Arm in arm, laughing and talking, we'd walk toward downtown, discussing our plans, or how their studies were going, or some point of Korean grammar I had a question about. After an hour we headed back to the jagrti, *our* new jagrti, and sprawled on the floor. Ripping open a package of unsold cookies and brewing up a pot of tea, we dug into a late night snack, a reward for our hard work.

I loved those people.

Dada S, my higher authority, swept into the region like a whirlwind every other month. This time I went to meet him at the airport. "How are things going? How are publications? What about the jagrti in Daegu?" He peppered me with questions on the ride into the city.

A charismatic man, his method of inspiring was to turn on the charm, which often succeeded in motivating margiis. But his occasional visits were not sufficient, I felt, for him to fully understand what was happening here. Invariably he came up with some new plan or switched people's responsibilities, creating problems for me after he left.

We sat down for a meeting that night. For months Dhruva had been planning to publish a book on yoga, but he'd gotten bogged down in the details, and had gotten nowhere. Dada was irked by the delay. "OK, OK, let's let Liilavati work on it," he said. I had to inform Dhruva that while his work on the project was appreciated, Liilavati would take over from here. Dada turned his charm on Liilavati, encouraging her to make this job a priority. The book was published, but hastily, and it contained many typos. And although Dhruva and Liilavati had been friends, cracks began to appear in their relationship.

I could see that from Dada S's perspective, not enough was happening in Korea. But this ignored the little successes, as well as the reality of the margiis' lives. These people were trying to fit their practices to their world, their family and work life, to live in their society as meditators. And while it's true that people sometimes needed to be prodded, the acharyas had to be careful not to push too much. I was beginning to see that the most successful acharyas took time to get to know the people they worked with, listen to them, and learn about their culture and psychology.

I liked and admired Dada S, and I also appreciated the fact that he never pressed me to raise money for projects in India. The acharya overseeing the work of the didis in Korea, on the other hand, was an Indian woman of authoritarian bent; her demands had driven a young German didi working in Seoul to resign from her posting.

Dada S was charged directly by Baba with the responsibility of growing AM in each of the East Asian countries. Not an easy task. He had to take risks. He had to think big. And things were going well under his supervision in other parts of the sector.

Although he sometimes seemed disconnected from the on-the-ground reality and I was sometimes frustrated by his intervention, I tried to respect Dada's advice. I tried, if it didn't create too many problems, to follow his orders. This was part of my commitment, too.

Seoul was a rapidly modernizing city, but I caught glimpses of old Korea, traditional Korea, like streaks of blue poking through a clouded sky. Seoul margiis were fond of hiking in the mountains and we sometimes spent the Sunday afternoons when I was in town up among the clouds, tracing paths through rugged hillsides on one of the many peaks surrounding the city. Though my health wasn't great, I found these hikes physically stimulating, if I didn't push beyond certain limits.

Hiking through Kwanak-San National Park one day, a group of five or six of us heard the strains of haunting music floating out from a hut in a nearby mountain fastness. The *klang klang* of cymbals and the guttural shouts could mean only one thing. A gutted pig's head teetered eerily on a pike outside the house. We asked a woman at the door if we could watch and she grunted in assent. So we crowded around the doorway and peered in.

The shaman, an elderly woman dressed in purple, twirled through the main room, smacking a large dried fish on the floor, people scurrying after her to clean it up. She grasped strands of colored cloth in her hand, and each participant of the ceremony held on to another end of a strand.

As the music picked up speed, the woman whirled with increasingly ecstatic abandon, calling out to the spirits, tangling the strands of cloth into an intricate weave. As the cymbals clanged at a higher pitch, the participants' faces grew heated with excitement. Finally, reaching some pinnacle, the shaman collapsed on the floor. The others, perhaps privy to a new inner awareness, leaned wearily against the wall.

Many Koreans, it seemed to me, nurtured a natural spiritual proclivity; they tended to embrace the mystical, and sometimes the messianic. Shamanic rituals were easy to come across in the older sectors of the city or in most rural villages. Many people strongly believed in traditional nativist ideologies, like *Tan Gun*, the creation myth, which claimed Korea would one day lead the world. The country also boasted the fastest-growing charismatic Christian population in the world. With what seemed a native intuitiveness and strong connection to nature, Koreans were open to all kinds of religious and spiritual practice. Small wonder that Rabindranath Tagore had dubbed the country "the light of the world."

Though I was learning a lot about the culture, in many ways I still felt an outsider. I wanted to get across to people with more clarity what AM was all about, a path that combined mysticism and rationality, the stark beauty of an organization that, despite its flaws, worked to uplift the downtrodden and spread a message of universal possibility.

But as I passed through the streets, shopped in stores, sat on the subway, or occasionally watched television, the fricative consonants of the Korean language exploded indirectly around me, leaving me dazed but none the wiser. I couldn't wrap my head around those lightning fast phrases, though I knew there were patterns there, like the '*hamnida*' at the end of sentences, which I learned was a standard verb ending, signifying the level of formality between speakers. But as for the rest, things were a bit of a blur. *Hankukmal,* the Korean language, seemed to consist of a series of larynx-wrenching vowels and harsh consonants designed to torment any Westerner foolish enough to try to speak it. Trying to follow a conversation I would look at people the way a dog looks at a person when he speaks, knowing something important was in the offing, but hearing only "Yah, yah, yah."

I had to invest some serious energy in learning the language.

My approach was haphazard at first. I kept a notebook of phrases learned, and constantly asked the margiis to explain themselves. Slowly, I picked a few things up. Narrowing in on the language from opposite extremes, my vocabulary became a kind of polar spread, at one end beginner's baby talk, at the other, philosophical terms I picked up in order to describe and teach the meditation process.

Breath calms the mind.
Where is bathroom?
Let your mind merge in Cosmic Consciousness.
How much that radish?

But I was determined to fill in the middle ground, and so I enrolled at Ewha Woman's University in Seoul; the Korean-as-second-language program there was open to foreigners of both sexes. I soon learned to read the alphabet and link together the Tinker Toy extensions of each letter. I grappled with the Subject-Object-Verb grammar, putting relationship, not action, first, which seemed appropriate for this society. I grew to appreciate the versatile adjectival nouns. Day by day my vocabulary grew. The day I understood a joke, I felt like dancing. I was repositioning myself as a person to be reckoned with in this society.

Our class practiced the stilted introductions, the obvious exchanges.

"Meeting you for the first time, it is good. I am a student."

"Meeting you, I am happy. I am a writer. What is your hometown?"

"My hometown is Portland. Where is your hometown?"

"My hometown is in Texas."

A number of Unification Church members were enrolled in the class, gathered here from around the world to learn Korean and work in the religion's headquarters. They were cliquish, sharing some Moon secret. But I got to know one woman after class. She had been matched with a husband in one of those mass weddings, and confided to me that she wasn't very happy with the results. Things hadn't turned out as she'd hoped; her husband was inattentive. We talked about spirituality and she fondly recalled reading *Autobiography of a Yogi* when she was younger.

I told her I knew it well, and after the next class session I lent her a copy from the jagrti so she could at least find some enjoyment in a nostalgic re-reading. It was instructive to get to know one of the Moonies individually. I still had the tendency to see them as somewhat deluded, but I was pursuing a way of life that many would find strange, so who was I to make judgments?

As for studying at a women's university, the brothers at the jagrti teased me mercilessly—a monk studying among thousands of beautiful coeds? "You are lucky," the Spanish student told me. "We can't even go onto that campus."

In fact, I was doing well at maintaining a dispassionate attitude in this arena. Ever since graduating from acharya training, I'd been successful with my celibate focus, a fact that surprised and pleased me. Occasionally, confronted on campus by a breathtaking beauty, my eye would stray, but because my daily practices strengthened the mind, it didn't stray for long. This life, its disciplines, its focus, its exercises aimed at redirecting one's energies, seemed to be working.

Besides, I was very busy and invested, struggling to get some things going. A vision of all the service AM could do here in the future sustained me. I was able to sum up my commitment in a common Korean phrase I learned early on:

Yaksok isayo.

I have a promise.

Goethe said, "Whatever you can do, or dream you can, begin it. Boldness has genius, power and magic in it. The moment one commits oneself, then Providence moves too." And indeed, things were beginning to percolate in the region, positive developments piling up.

A well-known translator of spiritual literature, someone who could help us navigate the Korean publishing world, came into my orbit. He was tall for a Korean, long hair tumbling down his back, and had become famous translating the books of Rajneesh into Korean. I invited him to a national retreat, and he showed up with his literary agent. They arrived at noon, when thirty Korean margiis were sitting in rows, meditating quietly, deeply, and sincerely. It was a beautiful sight. Afterwards he came up to me, impressed: "These people really know how to meditate."

A group of us in Seoul had begun regularly visiting a retirement home. We sang to the old folks, rubbed their shoulders, listened to their life stories, their memories as vivid to them as the trees outside their building. We also made sure they had sufficient warm clothing for the harsh winter soon to come. Whenever our little group arrived, though their faces were lined with care and age, these old people smiled. And we smiled back.

I was able to teach introductory meditation to quite a few people, and to teach advanced lessons to many of the older margiis. These lessons dealt with control of the breath, the strengthening of the cakras, and a technique known as *madhuvidya*, which helped one to see the sacred nature in everything. It was good to see people embracing sadhana in a heartfelt way.

Some of the margiis also began to come to me for personal advice. One young man was scheduled to enter the military for compulsory service after a few days. A slight, gentle person, unsuited for the rough life of boot camp, I remember him mostly for how he enjoyed poking fun at the Nancy and Sluggo cartoons printed in the English newspaper I received.

"Dada, I don't want to go," he said.

"Listen," I told him. "Be strong. Remember your spiritual focus. Be patient and see what you can learn from it." What else could I say? But I was glad he shared his fears with me. I was coming closer to many of these people.

Sometimes I had business downtown, and when demonstrations weren't exploding in the streets, I took the opportunity to explore. I wandered through Pagoda Park where old men sat in clusters playing "Go" and gathered around hawkers touting miracle cures for the complaints of the old. I sat outside the Myongdong cathedral, a place of sanctuary for radical activists, and did my noon sadhana. Despite all the financial and cultural struggles, I was happy.

Often I walked into the hills outside the city, where spring water bubbled up from deep in the earth, fresh and pure, water that was good for my health. (I heard recently that most of these springs have been closed, polluted by the black air wafting down the Korean peninsula from heavy industry in China). Often I came across ancestral grave mounds. There was no one there I knew.

One day I watched an old man fill his five-gallon jug, stuff it into his backpack and slip it onto his curved back. He exchanged greetings with an old woman striding up the hill, who had come to rinse out her cleaning rag. Perhaps she lived in one of the ramshackle houses nearby, with two or three rangy dogs leashed outside, and carrots and peppers in rows. She laughed, and humming to herself, continued on up the mountain.

I smiled at the exchange. It wasn't simply the physical dimensions of this land that filled me with elation, although those were striking enough—the high waters, forests of pine, craggy rock outcroppings, and spectacular views of ever-receding mountain ranges. Those things were all elevating and nurturing; but that landscape is charged now in my memory with the sense of purpose that I brought to it, the kindnesses of strangers-turned-friends, the feeling of being on an endless adventure, and the wonderful reversals of perspective afforded by settling into a culture that was as different as those pine-ringed lakes were from the flat prairies of Iowa I lived on as a boy.

This combination of things—stark beauty, true friendship, adventure, spiritual growth—led me to feel a contentment and a kind of maturity I had not known before.

Hiking up the granite-laced paths of Kwanak mountain, passing elderly climbers on the path, I couldn't help but appreciate their encouragement, as they chirruped in Korean, "*Sukohesumnida!*"

"Well done!"

Chapter Thirty-One

Ever since my days in Bangkok I'd become accustomed to receiving a fairly constant flow of inspiration. Stories flowed out of India about Baba's projects, his ideas, his songs, and his discourses. In the 1980's alone, he'd served up an impressive list of accomplishments: 5,000 Prabhat Samgiit songs. An expansions on Prout theory (such as the conceptualization of a "people's economy" related to how economics affected ordinary people). The social ideals of Neo-Humanism and Neo-Humanist education. The development of a number of botanical gardens. Lectures on philology and history. Books on Indian Tantric history. He had also overseen the creation of a network of schools, as well as a plethora of relief and development projects.

Recently, Baba had posited and discussed in detail a completely new field: the existence of a definitive subatomic link between matter and consciousness, which he termed *microvita*. This theory sent margii scientists into frenzied discussion mode.

This was not to mention the hundreds of small but transformative interactions he engaged in on a daily basis with people, spiritually uplifting interactions that made their way out of India in the form of "Baba stories."

I'd been in Korea for a year and a half, and in Asia for more than six. Now, again, came a new organizational emphasis. Baba was asking for model rural communities to be established in every region of the world. Like the little farm I'd visited in Batu Gajah, or the large model in India, Ananda Nagar; these rural intentional communities, Baba predicted, would link up and serve as a network of service and sustainability across the globe. In this light, he viewed them as important models for the future of the planet.

One thing I had learned—when our guru asked for something, we devotees were generally delighted to respond. This idea of wanting to please the guru was reinforced by stories from other traditions, such as the one about Milarepa, the yogi who lived in Tibet during the Middle Ages. Milarepa's guru asked him to build a house, and he did so. Then the teacher told him to tear it down and rebuild it in another location. He did so. This seemingly infuriating request happened several times. The requests, the story went, could be seen as a Tantric test, designed to exhaust Milarepa's karma. The idea was that tremendous physical and psychic clash "burned" Milarepa's samskaras, until he was pure enough to receive his guru's teachings.

Baba's requests might be seen in a similar light, though they usually were aimed at some concrete improvement in the world. It's true that karma yoga—serving others with an attitude of surrender—was, I had learned, a good way to grow spiritually. But the bottom line was, it made me happy to think about making him happy. Still, sometimes the request could seem awfully imposing.

When word came from the central office that Baba wanted a rural center in every region, I took it seriously. I sat with a few of the more experienced Korean margiis and we mapped out a plan. Then I began scrambling for money to buy land, contacting each of the margiis individually, explaining the project, and asking for donations. I also approached acquaintances. One day I went to see a wealthy woman to whom I occasionally taught English, hoping she'd come through in a big way. I brought Jiitendra along.

"You must be very busy," the woman asked, "asking so many people for little donations?"

"Yes…"

I was intent on asking for a million won, a lot of money, but Jiitendra was reluctant to translate this. *She won't…* He fidgeted. *How can you?* But I had to find the money somewhere, and so, putting aside the possibility that I might spoil this relationship, I pushed. Jiitendra squeaked out the request. The woman was polite, but got across to us in a roundabout way a definite refusal. Probably I had overstepped my bounds.

It didn't seem possible that we could collect enough money through donations. But occasionally I was surprised. A man who had previously taken little interest in our work, for example, donated a few thousand dollars from out of the blue. "Yeah, I heard about what you were doing, and it seemed like a good idea," he told me, unassumingly.

For several months all I, and a few others, thought about was how to find land, how to finance it. Korean land prices around this time were rocketing; the small country was in the grip of feverish land speculation. How could we possibly find an affordable parcel of land? The task was daunting.

Dada Shakti, the Argentinian monk I'd known in Tokyo, arrived for a visit, intent on helping with the land search. He had started the bakery in Taipei, and was considered a successful acharya, someone who could get things done, as well as a creative person, a painter. We traveled together to Jeonju. Shakti knew the search was not going well, and on the bus he scolded me, flexing his senior acharya muscles.

"You have to guide these people!"

I tried to look chastened, but I knew he wasn't really angry. He was just doing what he had to do as my supervisor. I took the point, and turning away, I smiled, because at that moment I felt very much in the game, part of the team. I was no longer the young inexperienced monk who needed to be treated with kid gloves. I was finding new strengths, and at ease enough within my own skin to accept this prodding.

And when we reached Jeonju, there was news.

"You have to see this land, Dada," one of the margiis excitedly told me. Though we'd just arrived, we wasted no time and set out again by bus into the countryside south of Jeonju. Soon we arrived at the spot.

It was beautiful. In front of us opened a flat expanse of rich soil, nestled among green plains, nudged by rice fields, and in the distance overshadowed by gently sloping mountains. We walked around it for some time, mucking about in the mud, then sat for meditation. It was a good place. We would try for it.

After weeks of going over the paperwork, Harideva and other senior margiis discussing the pros and cons, the ins and outs of land acquisition, and the acharyas reminding them that Baba himself was asking for this, the deal was finally sealed. With the help of earnings by a few acharyas from outside Korea, and donations from many local people, we were able to purchase several acres, not enough for larger-scale farming, but good enough for gardening. Good enough for now.

What a rush! Everyone involved felt the scope of the accomplishment. We'd taken a major step forward in the growth of AM in South Korea. As for me, I'd been working so hard on the project that I'd forgotten about everything else. It was only when we finalized the arrangements that I was able to relax. In the decompressing period afterwards, I had dinner with a margii couple in Jeonju. The woman happened to ask how old I was. I had to stop and think.

Then I realized. *Oh! Today is my birthday.* I was 28 years old.

One night back in Seoul I returned home from language class, ate some dinner, and almost immediately felt queasy. I went to lie down for a while, but soon felt feverish. Dhruva, who happened to be visiting, poked his head into my room, and his eyes went wide. Reflected in his face I saw the seriousness of my condition.

Once again, the liver problem had flared, and my health drained away from me as if a faucet had been opened. For days I lay in my room, very sick, my energy mirroring the pulses described in Chinese medicine: wiry, slippery, and elusive. Every action on my part took great effort. I vacillated on simple decisions until Jiitendra took to referring to me as "Dada Maybe."

After three weeks, my acute symptoms had mostly disappeared, and I wanted to get back to work. Harideva arranged for me to teach a yoga class at his Merchant Marine union center. There were lots of well-to-do men there who could help us financially, and with making contacts in a certain sector of society. I began to prepare for the class, but the day before it was to begin I called the whole thing off. I still felt too sick to take it on.

An acharya friend from Taipei came to visit and saw how tired I was.

"Do you want to go to Taiwan and rest for awhile?" he asked. It was a compassionate gesture, especially in this organization that held such great expectations for its workers. It touched me. But I myself had great expectations.

"I don't know, Dada. I guess I don't want to leave my post." He nodded. And I stayed on. Was my response heroic? Or foolish? Certainly it was self-sacrificing. I assumed that my health would eventually get better.

But I could no longer keep the pace I had set previously. Sitting and chatting with the margiis had to take the place of going out and starting three yoga classes or giving two philosophy seminars. I had to learn to be satisfied now with being, not so much with achieving. But a lesson seemed buried here: the little things, done with right motivation, could be as fulfilling as the grand visions.

Despairing for my health one day I went to my room and belted out kiirtan for an hour. Stirred by the intensity of my singing, the other brothers were pulled from their rooms to join me. We sang on with abandon, until bliss melted away all frustrations.

Even in the hardest moments something always occurred to shift my mood. A bit of grace—a kind word, inspiring passage discovered in a book, support from a friend, or an ecstatic shift of consciousness during meditation—was always forthcoming. I only needed to be patient. Change, I realized, always comes.

After all, there was something extraordinary about this Tantric path. And the jagrti in Daegu, site of so many struggles, home to those good students, made this realization manifest.

After our having occupied the Daegu jagrti for a year, the landlady suddenly and unexpectedly asked us to move out, saying she wanted to use the house herself. We had struggled so much to maintain the place that this came as a great disappointment. But there was nothing we could do. I came down to Daegu one weekend, and with one of the margiis, a gentle and committed young man named Shiilabadhra, set out looking for another house, stalking the streets in search of a 'for rent' sign. We walked all day and found no suitable place.

The next day, a sister named Parashakti called to say she had found the perfect new jagrti. We hopped a bus to meet her and when we got down, she escorted us to a large, second floor loft for rent. It was large enough for yoga classes and group meditation, yet there was something about it I didn't like. It fronted on a noisy street, for one thing. It just didn't feel right.

"I'm not sure this is the place for us," I told Parashakti. She'd been excited about the find, and became upset. We rode the bus back to the old jagrti in silence.

When we arrived, we found the landlady waiting for us. As soon as we entered the courtyard, she leapt up and began speaking animatedly in Korean, most of which I couldn't understand, but I knew something was up by the way Parashakti's eyebrows arched higher and her eyes grew wider as the landlady spoke. We all went into the house as the woman chattered on and on.

"What is it?" I asked finally.

"Well," Parashakti began, "She says she had a very strong dream last night, in which a man came to her and told her that it was important that we stayed here, in this house. The dream impressed her so much, she's decided to take only one room at the back, block it off from the rest of the house, and leave the rest to us." The landlady now glanced into our meditation hall, where a large photo of Baba rested on the table. She pointed at the photo and began speaking again, clearly excited.

"She says that's the man who appeared in her dream last night, and asks who he is!"

I glanced around at the others, registering the wonder that appeared on their faces. A wave of feeling washed over me.

Tell her he's someone very special.

CHAPTER THIRTY-TWO

Late autumn in Korea: the scent of pine in the air, a hint of brisk Siberian winds sweeping in reconnaissance gusts down the peninsula, binding North and South in chilly unity. Colors of maple dotted the ragged hills; roses appeared on the cheeks of uniformed school kids. The sweet potato man pushed his cart down the alley to the opening of the subway tunnel to get out of the wind. Apples and pears matured into fruition on the trees, and in the marketplace strings of brown dried persimmon dangled from shop eaves.

In December I flew to Taiwan to attend a conference. Afterwards, I was relaxing at the jagrti in Taipei with a few of the other monks. Dada M, a sweet and impish Italian monk, lay on the floor propped on his elbow.

"Hey, Alok! Why aren't you going to India this year to see Baba?"

I confessed to him the dismal state of my finances; there was no way I could afford a ticket to India. Besides, I had too many responsibilities in my region.

"Why think in terms of money?" he said, turning his big brown eyes on me. "You have a chance to see your guru, and nothing else should come in the way of that. How much longer is Baba going to be with us? We all have responsibilities, but think how much more inspired our work becomes after seeing him."

I appreciated his zeal, but the fact remained that I was broke.

M got up, stretched, and said he would talk to me later.

That evening he pulled me aside to say that a Taiwanese margii had agreed to loan me the money for a ticket. What could I say? I decided the situation in Seoul could get along without me for two weeks. I had been working hard, and I really, really wanted to see Baba. I told Dada I was touched, and that I accepted. He just grinned.

Since I was blacklisted in India, my adventurous plan was to fly to Kathmandu and enter India overland, at one of the small border checkposts in the foothills of the mountains, which by virtue of its obscurity would not be hooked up to the mainframe of the Indian immigration computer system, or so I'd been told.

My health, of course, was delicate. I'd recovered somewhat from the acute liver illness, but was still tired much of the time. But something about the prospect of travel, new scenery, and going to see Baba again promised energy, though I knew I would have to rest quite a bit along the way.

I awoke in the plane five thousand feet above the Himalayas. Shaking off my drowsiness I turned to peer out the tiny window and then gasped at the first view of those wondrous peaks awash in snow and moonlight. Massive folds of granite, undulating like giant paper fans, stretched on as far as I could see. These mountains were so much grander than any I'd encountered. Here I was, soaring above the highest point on our planet, close to the heavens, as our speck of a plane lost itself in contiguity. Perspective suddenly seemed to lose all meaning. We were simply adrift, inching across the face of infinity. I couldn't help being moved.

After my plane touched down, I stood on the back porch of the Kathmandu jagrti warming my hands in front of an ashcan, chatting with the local AM leader and a few others who were also traveling overland to India.

Some disheartening news had come. Baba was sick and had been hospitalized. DMC was postponed. Crestfallen, we mused about what this meant. The question of the moment, though, was whether we should proceed to India. Even if we couldn't see Baba, we could still spend time at Ananda Nagar, hang out with other margiis, be with our spiritual family. And perhaps Baba would surprise us. We had come this far; there was really no question of turning back. So we made plans to leave in the morning.

Next morning I located the bus headed for India in a downtown bazaar and hopped on, nestling in among passengers and piles of baggage. The bus was packed, boxes and bags shoved into every available space. I sat with my knees bent toward my chest. Though departure was set for 8 a.m., we sat and waited for two hours. Finally the driver arrived, grinning. Climbing through his door, he slipped a tape of Indian film music into the cassette player and we were off. Thick diesel smoke billowed in our wake as we lurched down the winding ravine roads, between the finger-like foothills of the Himalayas. We passed mud-daub houses, an occasional lamp burning in a shadowy window etching out a lonely tableau.

Arriving at the small wooden Indian immigration building on the border around six in the evening, the passengers stepped off and shuffled inside. Some of them, I noticed, slipped a few rupee notes to the officials. Perhaps I should have, too. There was, as I'd been told, no computer, but one official—not one of the crisply dressed authority-bearing men of New Delhi or Calcutta immigration but a sadder figure—dispiritedly ran his finger over a folded printout of pages several inches thick. It was the dreaded blacklist in hard copy form. But the list was too thick for him to go through at any length. All seemed to be in order. We reboarded the bus and settled in, waiting again for our dawdling driver. Ten minutes passed. Twenty. Where was that damned driver?

Suddenly one of the immigration men ran out of the building, climbed onto the bus, ran his eye over the passengers and... called out my name.

My heart lurched, then sank. The man had apparently continued to pore over the list and come across my name at the end of the printout. I thought about sliding lower in my seat and ignoring the summons, but knew that eventually I'd be identified. So, gathering my belongings and stumbling over the boxes piled in the aisle, I glared at the man, and while the rest of the passengers gawked, stepped off the bus and was escorted back into the office.

From there I watched my bus sail on into India, curious faces gazing at me through the dusty back window.

What now? What would they do with me? Would I go to jail? I had done nothing wrong. Still, I was a big catch. A margii trying to enter their country! The head of immigration was roused from his dinner at home. He was a strange man with crude digestion. Continually straining to pass gas, he uttered a little bark after each fart; his interrogation was punctuated with these disconcerting noises. Four or five rustic men now sat in a circle and glared at me.

"So." The chief fixed me with his best accusatory stare, and farted. "You engage in group sex?"

I laughed out loud.

"I don't even engage in regular sex."

His question, I guessed, was based on some backwater rumor related to spiritual groups outside the mainstream, combined with the idea that I was a hedonistic Westerner trying to sneak into their country.

I asked to go to the bathroom; a guard accompanied me around the back of the building to the latrine. In the dark corridor he grinned and asked me about life in America. I stood under a dim bulb in front of the cracked mirror and splashed water on my face, trying to steel my nerves.

When I returned to the main room, I found the chief had written in my passport, "This foreign national is banned from entering India as he is Ananda Margii." This was a mistake on his part, since it was technically illegal to deport me on those grounds, and such a written statement could be used as evidence against the Indian State in a court of law. But this knowledge was useless to me at the moment. After an hour or so of half-hearted intimidation, the chief waved his hands at me. "You go! You will not enter our country."

I was escorted back across the bridge to Nepal immigration by the same hapless guard. As we walked, I asked him, "Do you know what *dharma* is?" It was an idea that often gave me comfort. He nodded.

"This is against dharma."

The man shrugged.

I spent the night in a cheap motel room on the Nepal side of the border, resting and considering my options. Paint peeled from the walls and ceiling; the bed was lumpy and hard. I dozed, fitfully, the injustice of being turned back percolating through my consciousness.

As I tossed and turned, memories of Texas flashed on my dreamscape. I remembered the migrants who'd streamed across the river from Mexico by the thousands in search of work. The restaurant kitchens and landscaping fields of Austin flourished with their labor, but their situation was precarious: always peering over their shoulders, always on the lookout for "the man." The free movement of capital from one region to another was almost always protected, but never the free movement of people. This struck me as wrong.

I thought then about how much I'd changed in the last few years and about my family. How many ways I'd grown up while I was away from them. Those years of striving to organize a flux of unruly feelings, to channel my experiences into a manageable, sense-making course— my family wasn't familiar with that struggle. Like a river swelling and bursting its banks in seasons of too much rain, my personal struggles had, seven years earlier, overflowed. I went abroad seeking peace. And, yes, I had found it. I was now working at something important, trying to help people grow, trying to serve. I still had my struggles, and poor health certainly added to the challenges. But in a real way, I was a leader. Would they have understood any of this?

What a life! I could never have imagined it back in Texas. Perhaps it was all meant to be, my karma pulling me into this relationship with Baba, onto this path. Or perhaps it was just the way things played out, my good fortune to find a way of life that had healed and energized me, at least on a non-physical level. I was glad of where I had ended up.

But for now I really needed to think about what to do next. One option was simply to steal across into India at an unguarded spot along the border. I wasn't particularly concerned about the illegality of this. The ends did justify the means, I thought, especially since the blacklist of margiis was not recognized by the Indian court system. But without a valid entry stamp in my passport, I'd have to be constantly on the alert. Even a routine interaction with officials would reveal that I had no stamp and I'd likely be tossed in jail.

If I did enter India now, I'd be crossing over into something more than just another country. I'd be putting my dedication to seeing my teacher above all other considerations. It was another level of Tantric surrender, trusting that Baba would see me through any danger. Of course, who could say it wasn't my samskara to be arrested in India? But I didn't think so.

I wanted this trip to have its rightful conclusion. I wanted to be with my teacher and my friends at Ananda Nagar. I wanted to plug back in to the tremendous outlet of inspiration that being in that environment offered.

And so I made a decision. I wouldn't cross here, but instead return to Kathmandu, fortify myself at the jagrti, and take a bus to another border town, where, someone at the jagrti had mentioned, it was easier to pick your way across the border without going through immigration. Once I made this decision, I felt a sense of peace. In the morning I headed back to the Nepalese capital on a no less crowded or more punctual bus. And, after a day of rest, and a briefing on the best place to slip across, I set out again.

I was able to walk into India relatively easily at an unmonitored border site. I simply pulled a cotton shawl over my head to conceal my Western features and followed the crowd of locals who were intent on doing some shopping in another country as they made their way across the border. I was nervous, but things went smoothly. Then I caught a train and made my way to Calcutta.

I didn't get to see Baba on this trip, since he was still in the hospital, recovering from a heart attack. I didn't see him, but I felt him. Perhaps this prepared me for the future, when Baba would no longer be physically around. I could not comprehend such a time, and no one was worried that he would die now. And he did not, at least not just yet. But his body was seriously ill.

I enjoyed spending time with fellow sadhakas in Ananda Nagar, meditating, participating in organizational meetings. I learned several new Prabhat Samgiit songs, like this one:

The winter's fog is spent; a star blooms in the sky.
On the crest of a gentle southern breeze you appear, smiling softly.
The young leaves have shaken off their torpor; blossoms cover the dry branches.
A warm current threads the ocean, and you have arrived, bursting with affection.
To the sweet chirping of birds, nectar oozes from the ripe buds.
For your pleasure, I am lighting all the lamps.
Come to me, beautiful one, with marks of delight lining your eyes.
While a panoply of colors floods the earth, come into my expectant heart.

It was a cold winter in eastern India, but spring would be coming soon. Spring always came. After leaving Ananda Nagar and Calcutta, I made my way back toward Kathmandu following a slightly different trajectory. As I approached the border, I faced an uneasy night stretched out on a wooden bench in a frontier train station. In the morning I would ride a commuter train back into Nepal, where I was legal.

Exhausted from the rigors of the last two weeks, my body was on the verge of breakdown. But as kerosene lamps snuffed out one by one in the nearby village, I felt content. I gazed over the scattered houses and tangle of banyan trees and up at the sky filled with a lunar sliver and countless stars. I fell asleep repeating my mantra. In the morning I splashed a little water on my face from a rusty spigot in the bathroom, and as breakfast fire smoke began to show in the early light through the trees, sat for meditation.

Soon, the train arrived and began to load with people. Things were fairly loose here, citizens of the two countries moving back and forth across the border for work or trade, although I'd heard there was a perfunctory checkpoint a few miles on.

A man gripping one of the safety handles on the outside of the train advised me to push my way through the quivering mass of people and get inside.

"Sorry, excuse me, pardon me, sorry."

Perhaps because I was a foreigner, people made space, the single organism swallowing me into its cytoplasm like an exotic snack. I popped through the first bunch only to be engulfed by a denser crowd inside the train. It was still early, but the train was stuffy and warm. I made my way to a corner. A couple of guys took in the sight of me, exchanged a few words in Hindi, and burst out laughing.

The train shuddered and we were off. Some kilometers down the line, we were shunted onto a parallel track. I strained for a look out the window and saw an official in uniform and cap approach the train, preparing to board. I huddled further into the corner. I'd been assured they didn't check very closely, if at all. But maybe I'd been misinformed.

After all of this struggle, was I now going to be pulled off? My heart pounded.

Please let me go unnoticed. Please let me get through.

I'm not sure what happened next. Whether the crush of humanity stopped the official from investigating too closely, or this was simply a routine stop, I couldn't know. But our train lurched on; this time we were definitely in Nepal.

I had done it. Slipped through the seams. I let the breath flow out of my lungs in one long, steady stream. The plains of northeastern India lay behind me, as did Calcutta. Before me rose the foothills of Nepal, and then the mountains, stretching on forever, unchecked.

CHAPTER THIRTY-THREE

After returning to Seoul from Kathmandu, I slept for three or four days. Then I got back to work. I discovered that Jiitendra had let the bakery work slide and spent much of his time just lying around. He didn't want to meditate, didn't want to do anything. The discipline of the path, the constant expectation to be doing something good, seemed to be getting him down. Perhaps he was longing for his old bohemian lifestyle, wanting to run off and work on his art, or roam through the forest. He did disappear once for a week, without telling anyone where he was going. When he came back, I pulled him aside and we had a talk.

I wanted to convince him to get back "in the flow." Jiitendra had always marched to a different beat, but his help was invaluable at the jagrti. And he *was* a very spiritual person. But perhaps his way was different.

"Isn't being out in the woods, being free, enough?" he asked.

I looked into his eyes. "There's more," I said. "There's much more."

We stared at each other, me hoping he would see something in my eyes that would convince him to come back to work in the bakery, to come back to live in the jagrti, to keep meditating. Perhaps I should have let him do what he wanted to do; I knew he didn't respond well to discipline. But I needed his help. And I felt that he *could* find his place within this tradition, with a little adjustment.

Finally, he said, "Well. I better get to work then."

And for a while, he did.

That fall Korea was hit by torrential rain, and part of Seoul—a poorer part—lay devastated under floodwaters. Many people had to leave their homes. Inspired by the relief actions taken by AM when floods and typhoons hit other areas, the margiis and I decided to do something. We went to the market and collected donations of money, spending a whole day canvassing shopkeepers. People were eager to help. We bought boxes of food and blankets that we handed over to the Red Cross to distribute.

As it turns out, Baba, who was somewhat recuperated, had taken notice of the Korean flood in the news, and in Calcutta was asking whether we were doing anything to help. Dada Dharma happened to be attending the reporting for our sector in India at the time. Not knowing of our relief work, he told Baba that the Korean margiis were sure to be doing something. So when he called to relay Baba's interest in the disaster, I had a surprise for him.

"We've already been doing some work, Dada."

He was delighted. Though not, perhaps, as delighted as I was to learn that Baba was thinking about us.

Now more than ever, though, our financial situation was precarious. Bakery income, especially with Jiitendra flaking out a bit, was down. I needed to pay off the loan for my plane ticket to India. One possibility might help, something I'd been avoiding for most of my time in Korea. I had no other choice but to pursue it.

I sought out an English language academy not far from the jagrti. They needed native speakers and I quickly landed a job teaching a daily early morning class. Standing in front of the classroom, I introduced students to English language pop songs and discussed the plots of American movies that played in Seoul like *Dead Poets Society*. I urged the students to express their ideas about these cultural phenomena in this strange language the best they could.

I enjoyed the creativity it required, but the strain on my health was substantial. Rushing off early each morning and interacting with a room full of students was a steady drain on my energy. Not to mention that it took time away from other work.

But I needed the money, so I bit the bullet.

About this time I began considering a trip back to the States to legally change my name. This would allow me to get a new passport and enter India again without having to go through all the rigmarole. Once I had pulled together enough money, I began to plan the trip. I called my parents, whom I had not talked to for more than a year. They were relieved to hear from me.

"What happened to your voice?" my mother said. "You sound so different!" Was she hearing the accent of someone who had now lived abroad for seven years? The confident tones of someone who had found his niche in life? Or the tiredness, the sickness I now grappled with?

Most likely she was picking up on a lack of energy. My body, especially after this last trip to India, had become like a pen running out of ink, leaving only faint marks on the world around me. Perhaps, I thought, I would rest a bit while I was in the U. S. and try to improve my health.

I encouraged the margiis to carry on with things while I was gone.

One of them, startled, asked, "You're not coming back, Dada?"

"Of course I'm coming back. We have a lot of work to do here." *Yaksok isayo*: I have a promise.

I didn't know then that a great challenge was about to be laid out for me. That my life, my way of being, was about to face a test and that the results might alter everything I knew. Some might call it a Tantric test.

The day for my departure arrived. One sister helped me carry my bags to the bus stop. As the bus to the airport pulled up, I turned to her. I'm not sure what moved me to say what I did. She was, I knew, searching for something.

"Do something great, something noble, with your life," I said.

These would be the last words I spoke in Korea for five years.

PART FIVE — IOWA

Chapter Thirty-Four

Learn their logic, but notice
How its subtlety betrays
Their enormous simple grief;
Thus they shall teach you the ways
To doubt that you may believe.
　　　　　—W. H. Auden, *Atlantis*

My rusting Ford crept along the two-lane blacktop behind a farm trailer loaded high with yellow grain. I had driven out of the tabletop fields of central Iowa, and now, the closer I got to the Mississippi, the more curved the earth seemed to become. On my right a prairie graveyard slipped by, its granite headstones listing. Every few miles, century farmhouses floated in the lonely fields like satellite moons in space.

I was on my way to a Trappist monastery near Dubuque for a week's retreat, looking forward to a good rest and a good think. I'd been reading Thomas Merton again, impressed by his depth and desire to create dialogue between traditions of East and West.

The farm truck pulled onto a county road and vanished in a cloud of dust. I sped up, and a few minutes later made the turnoff to the abbey. Rising impressively out of the swell above a creek bed like a Chinese temple in the crook of a mountain, the monastery was both strangely out of place and neatly attuned to its environment.

Pulling into the parking lot I marvel at the building's humble magnificence. In the main office I met Brother Felix, a shy older man assigned to welcome the outside world into the contemplative mysteries of the abbey. He slid a schedule across the desk to me describing the seven daily "offices" or liturgical chantings, meal times, and a request to respect the silence. Then he guided me up the stairs to my room, a small neatly furnished cell overlooking a courtyard.

Through arched windows in corridors, I saw robed figures slip by, dreamlike.

The next morning, as the monks entered the chapel to recite their readings and chant their liturgies, I remained in my small room. I flipped open a travel-worn notebook containing my collection of Prabhat Samgiit songs and began to sing:

The winter's fog was spent, a star bloomed in the sky. On a gentle southern breeze, you came smiling softly.

I examined my conduct over the last couple of days for signs of the six fetters and the eight enemies. Anger and lust—Sometimes. Pride and fear—Not so much. Doubt—Certainly.

Then I crossed my legs into lotus pose, sat erect, closed my eyes, and performed the preliminary meditative exercise designed to disengage myself from the world while I focused my concentration.

On the far side of the building, the Trappists read from the Book of Matthew. I repeated my mantra and visualized myself becoming one with a vast underlying flow of consciousness. Neurotransmitters clicked in my brain like telegraph machines, seratonin on the rise.

I was drawn here because I thought they must speak some version of a language I understood, even if our syntax differed. This was a Western site of contemplation, of mysticism. I had spent the last seven years of my life on an Asian spiritual journey, and I longed to be in an environment vibrated by spiritual dedication.

Merton, the West's most eloquent contemporary spokesperson for the mystical life, put it this way, "It is in deep solitude and silence that I find the gentleness with which I can truly love."

These words and this environment struck a chord in me. For I read there, and saw in these monks, a reflection of what I'd been. I, too, had followed a shining sense of greater purpose across the earth like a golden grail in the sky. And yet, I wasn't sure where my life's purpose now was to be found.

After a nap I took a walk on the surrounding river valley farmland. The monastery maintained several hundred acres of farm and forest. These monks were pioneers in organic farming, but this land was off-limits to the public, so I walked across the road to another farmer's field. It was late afternoon and light danced across the soybean plants. The fields seemed somehow different from the Iowa of my childhood. Smaller, more defined, sadder.

They were much different, too, from the craggy hills of South Korea where I had not so long ago hiked regularly with friends. There the mountains ripped the terrain like giant teeth. In Iowa, the earth was comparatively flat. A Korean friend had been fascinated by the idea of a place where one could see the horizon stretching out in all directions. I had promised to send him a postcard.

Across a wide, open space stood a copse of fir trees, for which I headed. After ten minutes I was winded. I had overdone it; my heart was racing, my limbs sapped of energy. Darkness was settling in, quickened by an approaching phalanx of storm clouds as the sun shuttled low across the horizon. I shuffled back to the abbey and went to lie down in my room, hoping to conserve enough strength to attend vespers.

I was still sick, though I didn't really understand my illness. A great fatigue had settled, like fallout dust, over my being. In Asia my body had been invaded first by that mysterious infection that caused my foot to swell like a balloon for six weeks, then by Hepatitis, and finally by a platoon of parasites setting up camp in my intestines. The combined effect of these illnesses weighed me down, forcing me to stutter-step in the busy life I'd chosen. Some days in Seoul I'd had to stay in and sleep, putting off my traveling or teaching schedule. If I got in one or two good naps a day, I could manage. But soon I found myself wondering how long I could last.

The body...the *annamaya kosa*...what was the *sutra*? "The body is the outermost layer of the mind." To what extent one influenced the other I was not sure. But as if the physical process was mirrored in the mental sphere, I was assailed by doubts.

That night I had dinner with Jonathon, a student who was hoping to become a Jesuit priest. Food for visitors was not strictly vegetarian, but there were enough goodies from the monks' garden to make me happy—fresh beets, spinach greens, boiled potatoes, cottage cheese, homemade bread, and fresh pies, both rhubarb and strawberry.

Jonathon had taken part in an "associate's program" which allowed him to live the life of a Trappist for several weeks, and he told us a story from the other side of the monastic enclosure.

"At one meal, a novice stood up to read from the scripture, as happens every day. But driven slightly nutty by the never-changing routine, he looked fiercely around at the assembly and instead bellowed, 'Nothing ever happens in this God-forsaken place!' For a moment, everyone was stunned, then the place rocked with laughter, and the monk went on with his reading."

We laughed, charmed by the honesty of the novice's reaction. Then I told my meal companions a little bit about myself. "I lived in India for a while, pursuing a spiritual quest. I was a monk, too."

"Wow!" Jonathon said. "What an experience. Why did you come back?"

"Well, I got pretty sick," I told him. Though I knew that was only part of the story.

I probably seemed greatly changed to my family when I stepped off the Korean Air Lines flight in Dallas. Returning to the States after seven years, I certainly seemed changed to myself. My cultural bearings were a little off, the grocery store question of "paper or plastic" throwing me for a loop in Denver where I'd spent a few days. Physically, too, I was different, my style of dressing (when not in uniform) was now more utilitarian: trousers, simple shirt, non-leather sandals. Much thinner, my pants bobbed around my hips.

My family and I hugged, a little awkwardly, and made small talk. "How was your flight? You must be tired." We piled into my father's Ford sedan. As we drove toward my parents' home through the burgeoning suburbs of Dallas, I told them a little about my work in Korea, a litany of my accomplishments. I wasn't beyond seeking their approval.

"We've published several books on yoga in Korean," I said. "I'm studying Korean language at the university." I told them how we had just purchased land outside of Jeonju and hoped to build a center there.

"I've never done anything like it," I said, followed by a pause. "I'm enjoying this life," I said.

Again they were silent.

Although I knew I could probably never convey to my family the joy I felt in what I was doing, I'd thought they might understand a bit of my life. After all, they'd raised me to love God, to put others first, to do good, hadn't they? It was probably difficult for them not to see me more often, but I had hoped they would be proud of my work.

And in fact my mother seemed sympathetic. "Well, at least you're trying to help people," she said. I smiled at her.

But my father, it seemed, was driven to dissuade.

The next morning after I'd decompressed from the trip, Dad said to me, "Your mother and I are simply concerned about your wellbeing, son," adding, "We'd like you to meet some people who could help you...process your commitment."

Almost immediately, I knew what this was. My father had been in touch with some organization, a group of researchers who compiled information about spiritual groups that didn't line up with a certain outlook of what they thought a religion should be. This organization advised family members on how to facilitate an exit for their loved one.

I was taken aback. *What are they thinking? Don't they have any faith in me?* But also my thoughts cried out, *Baba, why are you putting me in this situation?*

Then, after some consideration, I decided to humor them. I had nothing to lose, I felt; I was secure in my life choice. The meeting might even be interesting, giving me insight into how my path was viewed from a more mainstream angle.

"OK." I shrugged. "I don't mind. But remember, I have a plane to catch Tuesday."

My father's relief was palpable.

We piled again into the family car and drove through rain-washed streets, oily puddles reflecting gray skies, into the industrial district of an anonymous suburb.

The two counselors were waiting for us at a motel. Joe, in snakeskin boots, jeans and finely tooled belt buckle, cultivated a carefully laidback image. Steve, more fastidious, had brought along fifteen shirts, well-tailored, bright, which hung in the closet in his room. Fifteen shirts for the two days he would be here? I supposed he thought he was holding a tempting array of colorful consumer choices out to me, assuming I was coming from a situation in which I'd been denied such choices. That, or he was a real clothes-freak. He was also, I learned over the course of the weekend, a disgruntled former member of AM.

They didn't strike me as sinister. But their agenda, I knew, was fixed. I eyed them warily. Preparing to get down to business, I closed my eyes, invoked my *second lesson* mantra, the one that helped you see everything as sacred, then folded my arms and began to watch the proceedings.

"There are orthodox religious traditions in India with their own validity," one of them began. "But what Andy is involved in is something else."

They talked on, comparing AM with Hinduism, a comparison that seemed specious since Anandamurti had distinguished AM's Tantric practice from the Vedic outlook of mainstream Hinduism from the outset. They talked about the problems with the organization, the controversies it had seen over the years. They talked about what they called the problematic nature of entrusting yourself to a guru. New religious groups such as mine, they said, too often demanded an unobtainable degree of purity from their members. Besides, AM must have used up all my money, and surely there was a lack of concern about my medical needs?

I listened. I didn't say much. I sensed that my family couldn't understand my relationship with Baba, or how remarkable he was. The meditation and other practices were beyond them, too, if they felt it was all "thought-control." This was disheartening. But why get bent out of shape trying to win them over? I must simply be the person I had become, and perhaps they would acknowledge something good there.

The criticism of using up my money seemed funny. I'd traveled all over Asia the past seven years, experiencing things I would never have had a chance to before coming abroad. I also didn't see validity in the point about my medical needs being ignored. It wasn't the organization's fault I'd gotten sick, and my supervisors had clearly tried to help me. The portrayal of AM as an unhealthy group didn't move me. I knew the organization had its problems, but I also knew that these were outweighed by what AM had to offer and accomplished.

And yet, maybe I *had* handled things poorly with my family. Maybe I should have kept more in touch with them. They couldn't help but worry, couldn't get a good understanding of what I was doing when they didn't hear from me for such long periods of time. The most grievous injury seemed to be that I had separated myself from them in becoming an acharya. There was no way around it—this was painful. Even in India, such a thing was difficult for parents to accept. In the West, there was even less context for it.

Some years later I talked with a good friend, a senior avadhuta who described to me how he had, many years before, handled leaving home to become an acharya. His parents were broken up about it; they asked him to meet with a psychiatrist. He did so, and during the meeting the psychiatrist came to understand that what my friend was doing was a noble thing, and he said so to the parents. Separation was part of the monk's life. But perhaps I could have dealt more openly.

Actually, my family knew very little about me. I had grown up while I was away from them. I was no longer the person I'd been, and that transformation seemed to be something to which they were blind. It was frustrating that we saw things so differently, that our perspectives on the benefit of my time abroad could be so divergent. It was as if two tectonic plates—my spiritual truth, and the emotional truth of my family's claims on me—were scraping and jolting against each other, and one seemed likely to buckle before the other, forming some new and unexpected landscape.

How many truths could there be in a given situation? And who, after all, got to say which truth took precedence?

As the afternoon wore on, the counselors dug and dished more dirt, everything they could come up with, from allegations of abuse of authority to cruelty, to at least one case of alleged violence. They argued that in the effort to achieve the mission's agenda, some AM members had acted in ways that were hurtful or heedless. I listened uneasily, yet these things didn't reflect the values of the organization I'd embraced. Yes, I could think of instances when people whom I knew had acted unmindfully. But I didn't think the problem of religious zeal running off the rails was a major problem in AM, if you looked at its history as a whole. In an organization of hundreds of thousands of people, you were bound to find a few trouble makers. Still, these isolated incidents had their reverberating effect. And if such things were all you heard about… well, I could understand why my folks were freaked out.

You had to acknowledge that Tantra could be dangerous. Andrew Harvey remarks on this in *A Journey in Ladakh,* declaring how the path of Tantra "has many temptations—to hedonism, to relish of worldly power.The man who can travel it successfully gains enlightenment in one lifetime." But knew it was not easy.

Anandamurti echoed this idea. Despite the nonsense a few of his followers may have gotten involved in, he was steady. "To tread the path of dharma," he wrote, "is to move on the razor's edge. Ordinary people… would like to know the way out, and the way out is devotion."

Devotion. Compassion. Love. It's what it all came down to. A great love was at the core of this path, a love that transformed faults and pettiness. My love for my guru, my love for God, kept me going. But what about love for my family, and consideration for their feelings?

I wanted them to accept my life choice. Or if they couldn't, I wanted to be at peace with that. Instead, I felt an obligation to appease them. It couldn't have been easy for them to have put this intervention thing together, to have participated in it, as misguided as I thought it was. They did it, I realized, out of love.

Another problem, spiraling back into our family's history, was that we had little experience in expressing our feelings to each other.

"Why aren't you reacting?" my father demanded at one point. "Why aren't you getting angry?"

"Look," I said. "This is your thing. I don't have to defend what I'm doing. Your minds seem to be made up already, anyway."

And then, something surprising happened. My father's shoulders fell, he slipped into his seat, and he put his hand to his eyes. He began to weep.

"We can't lose you!" he cried.

Oh, man. His words moved some lever of feeling inside me. Could I really be the compassionate being I claimed to be when I was causing my parents so much grief?

Perhaps the most important concern raised during this improbable family reunion was one with which I had yet to fully come to grips. On this trip I'd begun to realize how stubbornly recalcitrant my health really was. If I stayed in the U. S. a while longer, perhaps I would find the time and space needed to recover both my health and relationships.

My ticket to Korea burned a hole in my pocket: I was supposed to leave in a couple of days and I had to make a choice. Either return to Seoul and the life I had cultivated, with all its struggles, but its joys, too, a life that was shaping me into a person quite different from who I had been growing up, or remain here, at least for a while, and try to heal my stubborn body.

The counseling session lasted a day and a half. Once it was over, we returned to my parent's place. Exhausted, I holed up in my Dad's study and placed a call to the Seoul jagrti, speaking with an Indian dada there. The connection was fuzzy and we kept speaking over each other's words.

"Alok, is that you? Where are you?"

"I'm in America, Dada. I'm, yes,...in America. Listen, I'm going to be here a little longer, a few weeks maybe. Can you tell Dada S, and the margiis?"

"Yes, of course. Don't worry."

"OK, thank you, and...Namaskar."

"Namaskar." And we both hung up.

Chapter Thirty-Five

I stood in my childhood bedroom, arms linked behind my back, inching my torso to one side, then the other, breathing slowly. Bending forward, my hands lifted into the air above my head. I felt my spine elongating, stretching. This exercise, *karmasana,* was said to create energy.

Afterwards I lay on the floor, a blanket folded beneath my spine. My arms rested at my sides, the palms of my hands turned up. I felt tension in my shoulders, and my calves ached, so I tried to focus on those parts of my body, to release the stress accumulated there. The *savasana,* or corpse pose, is one of the most restorative poses, and I needed some restoration. But it also seemed appropriate that I was lying in a posture that imitated a dead body. To tell the truth, I felt as though something had died inside of me.

After a few days I went up to Iowa to stay with my sister and her family in Fort Dodge, a small conservative city in the north central part of the state. She'd generously invited me for a change of scenery. Away from my posting, away from other margiis, more than ever meditation served as grounding for me. I tried to not let my family's intervention upset my mental equilibrium too much. But it wasn't easy. I felt raw.

A visit to the doctor revealed the parasites occupying my gut, and they were soon blasted out of existence by a round of equally hard-core antibiotics. But something else was going on. Even after resting for two weeks, I still woke feeling exhausted. I had, I realized, felt just as tired for much of my time in Korea.

My sister and I struggled to find common ground. I think she assumed I would simply step smoothly back into American culture, let go of all my crazy yoga ideas. I couldn't tell her how much I was struggling.

One evening while Sue and her family were out, I left a cooking pot too long on the stove. When she returned, she found the pot soaking in the sink. "What happened?"

"Oh, yeah," I said, "I burned it." Something in my tone must have struck her.

"Don't acharyas apologize?" she said.

I sputtered. "You have no idea what acharyas do or don't do!" And stormed off to my room, a little overdramatically. Anger at my family for not believing in me, for not accepting my life choice, was churning a hole in my insides.

I wanted to think more about the questions that had been raised during the intervention. I went for walks in a nearby park, shuffling through the reddish leaves piling up under the trees, and sifting through memories of the previous seven years. There was no question that I had gained a degree of clarity through the practice. But when it came to some of the problems within the organization that the counselors had mentioned, it seemed there was a mystery here I couldn't yet solve. A thread, however slight, stuck out, creating a mismatched color in an otherwise beautiful fabric. It was likely that from time to time a few individuals in AM had been more interested in expanding their own power base than in spiritual development.

Of course, I didn't understand this when I was in Asia. And this demonstrated a weakness with the way AM explained itself, circling the wagons and not discussing problems. Something could be learned here about how groups, no matter how beautiful, how appealing, sometimes operated. Institutions in general tended to resist admitting to moral lapses. They tended to act to preserve themselves.

I kept thinking and reading. And eventually I came across an article in a major Indian magazine, *Hinduism Today*, which seemed to strike a fairly objective tone. "The early stages of [Sarkar's] organization's development were characterized by a zealous, high-profile and outspoken social/political posture which eventually churned a backlash of highly publicized conflict and controversy that has been very difficult to overcome. Only through arduous, unrelenting social service coupled with a carefully restructured public image, sustained over a number of years, has the Calcutta-based Guru quelled earlier animosities. Good will toward the movement is growing steadily as they overcome bad press with good works..."

I nodded and it went on, "Fiercely dedicated to certain political and social objectives in addition to their more contemplative endeavors, Ananda Margiis have fascinated and attracted a wide variety of people through the years. From quiet humanitarians and aspiring meditators in pursuit of the ultimate enlightenment to fiery radicals and political activists out to change the world, the ranks of Ananda Marga have swelled with a colorful kaleidoscope of individuals." That too seemed right.

Most spiritual movements, I mused, had their share of early missteps. When you slotted yourself into a system that required great discipline, you had to be sure you were doing it for the right reasons. It took me time to understand, too, that although meditation helped people to expand—to serve and to love more—that karma also ran deep.

There's a favorite line in a Saul Bellow novel. As I wrestled with some of these issues, I began to understand how true it rang: "Each of us has bitterness in his chosen thing."

A masseuse in this small city held weekly "healing circles." Like people at a party who discover they're from the same hometown, I was pulled toward those locals who embraced alternative spiritualities. This masseuse was a true psychic; at the first circle I attended, she touched my arm, and then described a scene from my sister's house—the upright string bass that stood in one corner—though she had never been there.

Three or four people showed up that night; one person lay on the massage table while the others sat and concentrated their positive energies on him or her. I was invited to go first. Climbing onto the table, I quickly became comfortable. The masseuse got things rolling, laying her hands on me.

She encouraged me to relax. And I did. Lying on her table, my mind soared into a vastness I had not felt for some time, part meditative stillness, part immeasurable relief at being understood by someone in this corner of the world. Her touch lifted me out of myself, gave me a taste again of what I most needed—an expanded view of self.

Afterwards she said that during the exercise she had felt something in me rise to the surface, a word: "Responsibility. My responsibility! Yours! His! Hers!"

And of course, this distillation of my inner state made sense. For what was it that had been asked of me, and what had I asked of others, if not to take more responsibility?

In the parking lot after the group broke up, she came up to me. "Are you all right?"

"Yes, I'm OK. Better than OK."

I asked her about her visions. "I didn't ask for them," she said, "didn't want them. I thought I was going crazy. But they came, and I had to come to terms with them. I had to accept it as a gift."

I nodded.

Chapter Thirty-Six

One night about a month after arriving back in the States I received a phone call that shattered my world. At first I couldn't believe what I was hearing.

Something had happened, something terrible. My master, great teacher, Tantric guru, inspiration to millions...

Baba had passed away.

Could this be? I called the office in New York and spoke with a stunned acharya who confirmed that, yes, Baba had left his body.

"What are we going to do now?" he cried.

The sky tonight is garlanded with stars. But darkness lingers in my mind. Whose absence, night and day, created this vast ocean of pain?

Putting down the phone, I made my way outside, my heart pounding, breath short. I looked up at the stars, pinpricks of light radiating over the world. The sky was bright, the Milky Way galaxy smeared across the heavens. But I felt no sense of wonder.

Instead, shock and sadness piled up in me, flotsam on a sea of sorrow. And a feeling of guilt. Here I was, back in the U. S., with all the old attachments and distractions, fumbling with my practices, and my teacher, who had done so much for the world was gone.

The flowers in the garden hold no fragrance. Without the moon, the sky turns sullen. Ice is not cold, honey seems tasteless.

Images flooded my mind, moments when my teacher had touched my heart. Baba standing in the driveway at Lake Gardens, singing Prabhat Samgiit songs. Baba walking in his garden, giving attention to a particular plant. I remembered listening to his weekly talks, crammed into the darshan hall with friends and fellow sadhakas. Because of him, I had experienced the thrill of a dedicated life. Because of him, I had learned how to love God.

My seven-year odyssey, an experience that had touched me so deeply, had seemed the truest thing I could do for myself and others. But it had all centered around Baba. And now, perhaps, it was unraveling.

Losing its tail, the peacock weeps and mopes, its vitality seeping away. The shuffling restless feet of dancing lovers have lost the beat.

I cried into the night.

CHAPTER THIRTY-SEVEN

In the winter of 1991, as U. S. Patriot missiles fell humming through the night on Baghdad, killing and maiming thousands of civilians, my own world continued to unspool around me. I was still reeling from Baba's death. And it seemed I might be leaving my acharyaship. My intractable health, the dispiritedness I felt at Baba's loss, the conflict with my family and the questions I had about the organization, all of this led me finally to understand what I was going to do, or rather, not do.

I would not return to Korea. I would try to figure out how to improve my health and see what else I could do in the world for the time being. I still loved the AM mission, but I needed time away.

It was not an easy step. Acharyas commit to their roles with the expectation that it is for life. But I had to be practical. My body was not up to the task.

I felt my sister's expectations weighing on me to become *normal* again. After a few months, though still very tired, I re-entered the work world and accepted a part-time job at a daily regional newspaper, first as librarian, then as reporter.

When the Iraq war started, I stood with the other staff reporters staring at the television, or pored over fresh AP copy describing the latest developments: Israelis huddling in Tel Aviv with gas masks; CNN reporters describing the siege from their Holiday Inn suites in downtown Baghdad; tank movements pocking the Iraqi desert. Some of my colleagues were shaken; others excited.

One of my duties at the paper included calling the families from our readership area who had military service members now in the Middle East. I was to ask them to send a photo of their son or daughter so that we could print it as part of a salute to the military. I spoke with many proud parents, all who saw their children's sacrifice in a patriotic light, and who were appreciative of our paper's coverage. This was hard work for me. Not only did I oppose the war, but I felt that my parents had not understood my own sacrifice.

I watched the American flags go up, read the editorials, stood at the newsroom window and viewed demonstrations in support of the war move down Main Street. I was anguished, the war seemed to stir up all the confusion and unresolved issues, the things I had tried to let go of when I took this job, when I decided to stay in the U. S. and try to fit in.

I still planted myself firmly outside the great surging patriotic swell. That part of my commitment—resistance to a kind of first-world hegemony—remained firm. But I watched my spiritual commitment erode somewhat. In Fort Dodge, I did not seem to understand anyone, and I would not let anyone try to understand me. One day I went for a long walk with my brother-in-law and tried to describe some of my struggles. He was a sympathetic listener. But his advice was simple: "Forget the past. Move on."

He could not know what he was asking me to do.

During that period of turmoil, my nights yielded images that bubbled up and washed over the scrim of my mind with astonishing vitality. In one rather pointed dream I was on a skiing trip with a number of margii friends, all of them zipping down the steepest slopes and flying carefree off the jumps into the air. I began to ski halfway down one of the steepest hills, then stopped myself just before plunging over the edge.

There was another intriguing dream: I'd been given a whole field to cultivate. I started turning the earth with a shovel, but my efforts were not deep enough. After some time, though, I was able to dig a very deep furrow, deep enough to stand in. A lot of garbage was collected there, and people were throwing in more. Someone wandered by and threw in a bed. I had the entire field left to do, but suddenly I glimpsed something shining beneath my shovel. I scraped the dirt away and realized that there were polished wooden planks, a very real structure buried underneath this field. The dream seemed a confirmation that, beneath all the garbage our minds took in, there existed something, deep down, which was strong and true.

Another dream cast a warm glow over my day. In this one, my mother came to me and said, "It must really be hard, when you believe in something so deeply, and someone tries to take it away from you."

All of these dreams hinted, directly or indirectly, at the depth of my experience in Asia, and the traumatic grief I felt in leaving that life behind. It would just take some time to feel normal again, if normal were indeed possible. Or desirable. What I sought was a sense of integration, of taking all that I knew and had experienced, and fitting it to the world I lived in now, this strange world where I had grown up.

Finally, one night I had this beautiful vision: I was in a jagrti, talking with others about why Baba's ideas hadn't yet been implemented in the world on a larger scale. We discovered a hither-to unknown room, with a wonderful heart-shaped surprise—packaged love, really—inside. One man said, as if realizing something, "Well, of course! First you have to get inside the room, then all these incredible ideas are listed on a parchment there and you have to copy them down." He demonstrated by writing in huge scrawling letters like a child, taking up one page with just a few words.

I lay awake a long time, thinking about this dream. The implication I drew was this—we didn't yet have the skills, the spiritual and moral stature to assimilate all the amazing gifts Baba had given us. It would take more time.

To my surprise I discovered that several margii families were living in Iowa. After getting in touch with them, I began attending group meditations. Their friendship was a breath of fresh air; they offered a way to reconnect and a sense of support. With their encouragement, I decided to attend a week-long summer retreat at an AM center in southern Missouri. A Bengali family from Iowa City offered me a ride down; it was an eight hour drive, and we stopped and picnicked along the way. Their eight year old son ran among the gravestones in the cemetery next to the park where we ate, and we stretched out in the sun, chatting comfortably about India, about our lives.

I knew very few people at the retreat—after all, I had lived most of my margii life in Asia. But joining in with 300 others on the kiirtan and meditation, I began to feel at home. The side of myself that I had questioned, put on hold, for the past year, was given free rein to express itself. Like me, these American margiis were still dealing with Baba's death. Conversations revolved around where a person had been when Baba died, and how they felt the organization was doing in this post-Baba era.

"I was stunned," one brother told me. "I thought, how can things possibly go on? But, of course, all we can do is continue to surrender, and do the work." The important thing, he said, was the ideology Baba had left behind. Playing midwife to these ideas, to a new spirit, or an old spirit newly expressed, was what we had to focus on now.

Although his passing was a great shock for his followers, I learned that a few days before his death Baba had recited a couplet by a famous Indian poet. "When I came into this world," he quoted, "I cried, and the

world laughed. Now that I am leaving it, I smile, and the world cries."
He had clearly known it was time.

One morning at the retreat center I entered a room set aside for
Baba to stay in, if he were ever to have visited the U. S. The room was
now used only for meditation and had a special vibration. Opening the
door, I was hit by a wave, a radiated spiritual energy. Several people
were sitting there doing their meditation. At the front sat a larger-than-
life sized photo of our guru. I sat down, crossed my legs, closed my
eyes, and immediately felt my mind dive into some hidden recess of
concentration. I enjoyed the meditation there tremendously. A little later,
drifting in a beautiful flow, I opened my eyes and glanced at my watch,
expecting maybe half an hour to have passed. Three hours had slipped
by in that blissful state.

Still, the conflict that had been kindled in Texas sputtered on
inside of me, and shaped some of the conversations I had at the retreat.
I ran into a British dada I'd known in Calcutta, someone who worked
hard at being sensible and non-dogmatic. We rowed a little boat out
onto the pond bordering the campus. As we bobbed on the water, I
expressed to him some of the concerns I had. That there seemed little
scope to express one's emotions in AM. That there was sometimes a
tendency toward rigidity. That we needed to work more with other
people of good will, and not think that we alone had all the answers.

"Yes," he agreed with a smile. He dipped the oars into the water
and we watched the water ripple in the sunlight. "We need to work on
all these issues more." It was reassuring to hear him say so, and I realized
that many people were thinking along the same lines now, in this era
when we were having to figure out how to conduct things on our own.
Not that Baba had allowed such things to take place; rather, that because
of the incredible Tantric urgency we'd experienced during his time, some
things had gotten pushed to the wayside. His absence now offered us
time and space to deal with this.

AM was a young organization, only fifty years old. Reflecting
the sense of speed and pressure Baba had leveraged, there seemed within
it an intense distillation of every kind of human spiritual endeavor—the
mystical experience, the selfless service, the communal fraternity, but
also, sometimes the dogmatism or even fanaticism. All the promise and
the all problems, too. But maybe the problems were part of the Tantric
package.

Beyond these discussions I received some compassionate advice.
"Take care of yourself," one sister, a former didi, told me. "No one can
say anything about you leaving your acharyaship. Love God and go on."

And this came from a jolly African dada: "Enjoy your life. Why feel guilty or worry? Otherwise, what's the point?"

I attended the workshops and classes, but my mind drifted elsewhere. Something was building inside of me. On the fourth day of the retreat, I wandered off for a walk in the woods. And there, amidst the cottonwoods, with armadillos and foxes scattering at the sound of my footfall, I began to feel some release. Alone in the forest, something began to be knocked loose. Something began to give.

Standing in a clearing, the frustrations of the past year tumbled out. I yelled at my father, for not being there for me as a boy, for trying to pull me out of a path that had given me so much. I yelled at Baba, for leaving. I yelled at those who had done stupid things in the name of this organization. As tears rolled down my cheeks, I raged at them all.

Slumping against a cottonwood tree, in a forest of the Missouri Ozarks, the very center of the North American continent, my voice echoed up through the trees and into the blue sky. I let everything out, and I began to breathe freely.

CHAPTER THIRTY-EIGHT

Having been offered a reporter's position at the newspaper in Fort Dodge, I gave it a try. I loved the work, but scrambled to find the energy to fulfill my duties. At lunchtime I ate a sandwich, then napped for an hour in the break room. When I went to another town to cover a story, I often pulled over on the side of the road and slept in my car. I told myself everything would work out, that my health would surely improve.

But after working for some months at the newspaper, I realized a full-time job was beyond me. I left and settled instead for a part-time gig at the local public radio station. On weekends, I was alone in the dimly lit station, the glowing lights of the control panel casting a faint glow around the room. I set an alarm clock, lay a blanket on the floor of the control booth, and slept. Five minutes before the top of the hour, I popped up, turned up the microphone, mustered my strength, and for sixty seconds tried to sound fresh and engaging as I read the weather, station identification, and upcoming programs. Then I went back to sleep.

Not long later I decided to move to Iowa City to finish my undergraduate degree at the University of Iowa. It was a big change. Though a fairly small city, under 100,000, Iowa City glowed with the lights of literature and the arts, hummed with the buzz of international students and scholars, radiated with liberal political views. Though I had studied English at Texas, my time abroad had generated an interest in learning more about culture; I set about slowly earning a degree in anthropology.

It was in Iowa City that I finally got a handle on what was going on with my health. In the bright offices of Dr. Zuhair Ballas, chief immunologist at the University of Iowa Hospital, I underwent a series of tests. Dr. Ballas was an eminently cheerful man, and seeing him always made me feel better.

On one visit he breezed into the office with his attending resident.

"So, how are you doing today, hmmmm? Read any good books lately?"

The last time I was here, blood had streamed out of my forearm into a series of tubes. It seemed a fair exchange—give us your precious fluids, we'll try to find out what's wrong with you. Dr. Ballas asked if I'd been following the modest exercise regime we'd chalked out—20-minute walks three times a week.

"Don't overdo it," he advised. "You know what can happen."

I did know—a common scenario was that on days when I had some energy, I tried to squeeze in too many activities and ended up paying for it.

"Take a look at this." He offered a pamphlet.

What is Chronic Fatigue Immune Dysfunction Syndrome? CFIDS is a serious and complex illness that affects many different body systems. CFIDS can last many years. Symptoms include unremitting fatigue; sleep disorder; muscle pain; impairment in concentration; headaches; post-exertional malaise.

What's in a name? Strangely, a measure of relief. Even though Dr. Ballas, and his retinue, and all he stood for, could offer no real cures, classifying my illness granted it some legitimacy. Though I might not have felt any better, it helped to know why I didn't feel any better. After several years of being on a hunt for the missing puzzle piece which would explain my illness, being referred from doctor to doctor, enduring the shrugs, the skepticism, or the suggestion that I was simply depressed, my faith in Western medicine had fairly dissipated. It was good now to at least receive some acknowledgment of my illness.

Still, I knew that here in the West, people tended to view the body in Cartesian terms: parts meshed together as in a great calibrated instrument, and the cure of disease was simply a matter of replacing the broken parts, or suppressing the symptoms of breakdown. But this was an incomplete model. Illness might in part be mechanical breakdown, but it was also something larger and more mysterious, something tied to energy and spirit. Even though my illness was now named, I knew that CFIDS was simply an umbrella term covering a range of symptoms, and that it didn't really begin to describe all that was happening with me.

In Asia, I'd been committed to a great ideal, and that had helped generate a certain amount of energy. Though I was often exhausted in Korea, having important work to do kept a level of energy flowing through me. Now that was harder to find.

And a question that had lain dormant under the activity of the last few years began to rise: If Tantra was about marshalling your energy and throwing yourself into work without reservation, what happened when that energy became severely limited? Was there room on this path for accepting fragility as an integral part of the human condition? Might Tantra be not only about an expansion of consciousness, but also, at least in terms of the body, about understanding that there were times of contraction, too, times to offer a compassionate embrace to the suffering of oneself and others?

Of course. It had always been so, even though I may not always have focused on this aspect. The practices of Tantra were geared toward all-round growth, healing and service.

I would remember this.

Chapter Thirty-Nine

Our plane banked over the craggy teeth of the Kwanak mountain range, which jutted into the sky as if to devour invaders. Didn't I hike that particular peak once? Wasn't that the national park where I stumbled upon a spinning shaman conjuring wealth and good luck by smacking a dried fish on the ground? Six years had slipped by since the late 1980's, when I'd spent several dramatic seasons on the land below. Flying into Kimpo now my mind was colored with a vibrant hue of memory. I knew that I was not the man I'd been before.

South Korea was still technically at war with the North, and the bulky flak-jacketed armed guards I'd remembered on every street corner still patrolled the airport terminal walkways. Chun Doo Hwan, tyrant in a long line of dictators stretching back to post World War II-liberation, no longer ruled. Stoked by the democratic breezes that inspired the overthrow of so many Asian dictators around the same time, South Korea faced a social and political sea change. The breeze had whipped up into a strong headwind, closing over the chilly strongman political model of the past, and chasing it north. Now came the hard work of coming to terms with the lapses and excesses of former rulers. A chilling series of construction disasters plagued the country. Just the other day, a shoddily built high-rise constructed during the earlier regime in one of the ritzier sections of Seoul had collapsed into rubble, imploding in a horrific reproach.

During the teargas-soaked years of 1989-90, I'd been Regional Secretary for Ananda Marga here. I'd been young, in a country where everyone was neatly slotted into a hierarchy of age relationship and obligation. Given more time, I think I might have integrated my personality more fully into the contours of that situation.

I'd made friendships, but they were circumscribed by my position; I'd been encouraged to inculcate a certain personal restraint, not mix too much with others, especially with women. I had struggled to manage things, especially financially, to keep our centers and projects running. And yet, a certain beauty, the nobility of a complete commitment, had infused the work.

And now I was back, ostensibly on a research grant to look at Chinese medicine in Korea from a cultural angle, an honor's project for my university degree in anthropology. But a sense of unfinished business, a longing to reconnect with that former life, drove me. I was to stay with a Korean family, an arrangement made by a stateside friend, but I also planned to meet up with many old margii friends.

My host family—widowed mother, grandmother, and three sons—lived in a small apartment on the outer ring of one of the concentric suburbs radiating for miles beyond the city of Seoul. Duk Jun, the oldest son, ruled the roost. On my first day here, as we were getting to know one another, he calmly commanded his younger brother to bring tea, and the brother responded unhesitatingly, comfortable with the role of supporting actor.

Duk Jun told me about being thrown in prison for six months during the dictatorship. He was charged with violating the National Security Law for organizing a group of factory workers. "I really did nothing," he said, "just talked to a few labor people. But one day a group of government men jumped on me, and then I was in jail." Once again, a story of government abuse. As we talked, his mother brought out dish after dish of extraordinary Korean food and nervously asked Duk Jun not to talk about those days. "Eat, eat," she encouraged.

The grandmother was 90, her face a raisin. She came from another era and spent most of her day staring out the window at the other apartments in the complex, or sitting in front of the TV. When a program about traditional farming came on, however, she became animated.

"I used to work like that," she said, pointing, and grinning her toothless grin.

Harideva, the president of AM in Korea was still around! Now in his late 60's, he had taken up running marathons. He was still kind, still given to sentimentality. We arranged to meet at a downtown hotel, and when I entered the room, he called out to me, "Dadaji!" using the old term of respect with its affectionate suffix. We embraced.

"How are you?" I said. "Please don't call me Dada anymore. I'm no longer a Dada."

"OK, Dadaji."

We sipped tea, and gazed into each other's faces.

"We miss you very much here. We had many good times together. Many people from those days left and joined another meditation group." He saw my disappointment.

"But many are still here. You worked hard." We sat and smiled at each other, he the former leader of the Korean margiis, me a former acharya tasked with helping AM grow in Korea. Memories of our time together leapt to mind—visiting the old folks' home, organizing retreats, walking in the mountains.

"Do you remember when we visited India together and I ran out of money, you helped me out, gave me money? I want to repay this debt, Dadaji." Suddenly he was pulling his wallet out of his pocket and flourishing 20,000 won.

"You don't have to do this."

"I want to," he said, and tucked the bill into my shirt pocket. "Have you come back to stay?"

The road to Jeonju ran through gorgeous territory, winding past hills with deep pine forests before emptying into the central plains. The bus passed a village with a bright carpet of red chilis laid on the road to dry. It was near here that AM had purchased the land for a retreat center.

An unknown woman greeted me on the bus. I thought it a fluke, but when we both got off at the last stop, I realized she was also going to the center. And I thought, in a moment of pride, she's coming here to this place, this place that I helped arrange. It was, as I'd remembered, a beautiful site, nestled in the crook of mountains. Stepping off the bus I was struck by the startling colors of spring, the winds of freshest air. A stream burbled past the bus stop. Nearby were a few houses in rustic country style, with curved tile roofs, bales of straw stacked against the walls, a stooped *harmoni* grandmother sweeping a porch.

Swinging open the gate to our land, I saw for the first time the house that had been constructed there— large, clean, and beautiful. Glass windows opened onto the landscape so that sitting in the hall one seemed almost to merge with the mountains.

Twenty people were here for a retreat this weekend, many of whom I knew. Over lunch I sat with some old friends; they chattered in Korean, and I followed along as best I could. One sister heard that I planned to spend a few days in Jeonju. "Good, Dada," she said.

I was feeling happy, but also, on some level, regretful, perhaps ashamed, that I had left my responsibilities here.

Now a little boy toddled up and stood next to me.

"Who's this?"

"It's Arjuna, Dada." The boy climbed into my lap, unafraid of this foreigner, as if some mysterious connection bound us. How strange. Six years ago I'd presided over the baby-naming ceremony for this boy— I'd given him his spiritual name. Now he seemed pulled to be near me. The boy ran his chubby fingers through my beard. I laid my hand on his head and smiled.

I skipped the afternoon program, and instead strolled the land, jumping lightly over the stream and mucking through the mud, inspecting the garden, climbing up into the hills and stumbling across a country graveyard, a clearing neatly pruned and raked amidst the tangle of forest. After an hour of wandering, I returned to the center where meetings were still going on in the main hall.

Perusing the books in the retreat center library, I pulled one off the shelf, opened it to the first page, and received a shock. There, inscribed on the frontispiece, in my scrawling hand, was my former name, "Ac. Aloka Brc." This had been *my* book, but when I was a different person. A sudden surge of emotion, of nostalgia, and of love for this spiritual path poured over me. I felt an opening, and at the same time, a sense of vertigo, as if I'd fallen away from something important. What was I doing with my life now? Running here and there, thinking about women.

Pulling this book off the shelf had pried open a door, and I peered through it, down a line into the future, trying to discern who I might have become. Perhaps I was grieving a little for a lost future self, for what I might have become had I remained an acharya: a dynamic worker and teacher, purposeful and focused, with enough experience under my belt to remain unflappable in any circumstance. My successor as RS Seoul had spent four years here, then been transferred to Berlin. Perhaps I, too, would have accepted a posting in another part of the world, another step in maturity in my organizational life.

But I'd taken another path.

From the retreat center I called my old friend, Om Karnath. He was at his country home for the weekend, at some ceremony honoring his ancestors.

"Do you know who this is?" I asked in purposefully stilted Korean, an old standard joke between us.

"Dada Alok? Where are you, in America?"

"No, I'm here in Korea, in Jeonju."

"Really? Wow! OK, can you stay there? I'll be there tomorrow." I hung up the phone and smiled. That he would drop everything and jump on a bus to Jeonju to see me meant a lot.

The next day he arrived, and we strolled on the muddy roads surrounding the mountain together. "I remember an incident about you, Dada."

"Don't call me Dada."

"When we were at Chi-san, in Daegu, walking down the mountain. You had been sick. On top of that, as we walked, you slipped and fell on some rocks and cut your leg. Then you said, 'Oh God, what *is* my karma!'"

He laughed and looked into my eyes.

"It was very honest and very funny."

After the other retreat attendees had left for home we were alone together. Over lunch, we talked about women and marriage.

"I would like to marry, now that I'm no longer a monk," I said.

He smiled. "Wow, I like talking freely with you like this. Before, we could not talk about such things."

Conversation turned to our families. I told him that there had been times when I had not gotten along well with my parents.

"You should be patient and accepting," he offered. But his words hung in the air, and the situation seemed strange, as if our roles had been reversed. Before, he had been a young college student, turning to me for advice. Now, he was a budding businessman, with an assuredness about him. The shift affected me. I grew shy, and there was an awkward pause in the conversation. For a while, we were not sure who this other person was.

Back in Seoul, I made contact with an old friend, now a graduate student in traditional medicine at Kyunghee University. He set me up with some research related to my project and also introduced me to a professor who had been looking for someone to help him write a book in English. In exchange for a room near the university, I met with the professor twice a week and helped shape his words. It was better for my health not to have to travel so much. So I left Duk Jun's place, his family tearfully seeing me off, and moved into the room, which happened to be near the home of a woman named Rosa.

Rosa had been a margii when I was posted here, but was no longer active in AM. She told me she just wanted to do her own thing, and not be tied to any group. I visited her studio one day and watched neighborhood children plunk Bach minuets on the piano under her patient guidance. In the corner a tiny girl with an angelic face practiced her scales, little fingers struggling to stretch over the keys. Sitting there listening to this simple music, I had a momentary intuition—what a wonderful life this was; how many possibilities there were in the world!

One weekend Rosa and I drove toward the DMZ to visit a Buddhist temple. *Gun-in*, soldiers, stood at attention everywhere. We strolled up the paved trail of the mountain and located the temple with its huge wooden, colorful Buddha. Inside we sat for a long meditation. When we'd finished, it had become quite cold and I was feeling exhausted. The resident monk invited us in to his room, heated by *undol*, that old fire-under-the-house method, to have some tea. There he told us stories about "holy fool" monks in Korean history. These stories strained Rosa's ability to translate, but I got the gist of them—it was better to *experience* "one-mind" than to talk about it.

Saying goodbye to the monk, we walked back down toward the car. It was a long walk, and I stopped next to a flowing brook to rest. Listening to the water gurgle beneath the ice sheathe, we sat in silence. Then she slipped her hand into mine and we headed back down the mountain.

A week or so before I was to leave Korea I spent another weekend on the land at Jeonju. There was a brother there who knew me, who said I had taught him meditation back when he was in the army, but for the life of me I couldn't place him. He was a strong young man, a leader, and had dedicated himself to the work of Ananda Marga in Jeonju, teaching yoga in town, organizing vegetarian cooking classes, and overseeing the growth of the retreat center. I was touched and happy to see such a strong margii. He clearly had respect for me, and yet I couldn't remember him.

We worked together in the garden, which looked great, full of tiny sprouts, a few early full-grown vegetables. There were plenty of weeds to be pulled. The sun arced across the sky and began to edge over the top of the mountain to the west. We worked in silence for a while.

Then something interesting happened. The brother pointed out some plants which, he said, came from America: beets and lettuce. And a feeling of déjà-vu washed over me. Suddenly, I realized that these plants had grown from the seeds I had sent to Korea from the U. S. five years ago, on the eve of my leaving my acharyaship. They were seeds I had planned to see put into the ground, before my own world turned upside down.

Someone had planted these seeds, and they had borne fruit.

EPILOGUE

A spring evening settles over the Iowa City skyline. I gaze out the window of my second story apartment, across the lawn to the garden, where just last week I spaded warm black soil, crumbled the clumps with my fingers, then broke free the roots from the potted Big Boy tomatoes, jalapenos, sweet smelling basil, lavender, oregano and lemongrass, placed the plants into the Iowa earth and hoed the excess soil around them. In my mind I was repeating the mantra for blessing, hoping these plants would do well this summer.

Some things are simple. This garden, for instance. And the vegetable stir-fry sizzling in the pan on the stove, while my aging black Labrador, Pete, noses at my feet for dropped ingredients.

Some things are more complicated. And some things take years to understand.

I see what happened after my return to the U. S. as a Tantric test, one that shifted my relationship to my path from uncritical acceptance to a more mature and complex commitment. Many of my questions have melted away in the face of devotion. But reason, I acknowledge, has its place, too.

It's easier to reflect on these things with the advantage of twenty years of hindsight. I write now with more compassion for that younger self, for my family. I wish I'd understood then about AM what I've come to understand now—that in an organization of this size, you always find a few troublemakers. People do stupid things.

Although I reconnected with and recommitted to the AM mission as a margii, not an acharya, it was a part of my life that I didn't share with my family. I did write my parents a letter not long after I decided to stay in the U. S., expressing my anger, but such was the emotional disconnect between us, especially on this issue, that no one ever brought it up again.

The simmering anger I felt dissipated, though, until after a few years it had all but disappeared. I was living an ordinary life, one disrupted by health concerns, but one that my family could appreciate—studying, teaching, doing community work—while continuing to do my sadhana, hang out with margii friends, go to retreats, and work on AM projects.

It was at Christmas, especially, that my family connected. Each year we gathered at my sister's home for the opening of presents. She worked hard to prepare a big meal, and there was much joking and talking around the dinner table as we enjoyed the food. Afterwards, I had time for a long afternoon nap in the guest room while my nieces and nephew watched *A Christmas Story* in the den.

After waking, I would sit for meditation for a few minutes. And then, eager to rejoin my family, I wandered downstairs past the wrapping paper detritus of the day, to where everyone was gathered, a feeling of joy spreading inside of me.

Consciousness, I understand from my study of yogic philosophy, expresses itself in a curved wave pattern, a flow of peaks and valleys. And of course, life itself is full of ups and downs, a fact my practice has helped me to accept with equanimity, especially as the dance of the ideal and the practical spun like a mobius strip in my mind for a few years after I returned to this country. My goal as a spiritual aspirant is to straighten out some of those curves—to increase the wavelength of my own mental waves, moving them closer to the infinite—and also to serve, to help others deal with the trying circumstances of life.

I'm reminded of these oppositions, sometimes, when I enjoy the songs of my teacher, the soaring highs and lows, piano to fortissimo, of Prabhat Samgiit. I still love to sing those songs, and even made a recording of some of my favorites. I often think about how fortunate I was to have been around while this extraordinary person was alive. A couplet of his lyrics ring through my head:

Your cosmic play is endless, beyond happiness and sadness.

In recent years, after Baba's passing, I watched a split occur within AM. The organization split into two, then three, factions. It was heart-wrenching to see the beautiful movement Baba created facing trying times. Much of the conflict seemed to be rooted in struggles for power. The solution, of course, lies in getting back to basics. More service.

More kiirtan and more sadhana. More rationality. And more selfless love, the heart of yoga.

More than ever I've come to understand that spiritual discipline aims not at creating a finished form, a fixed structure, the brittle shell of belief. Rather, it's the art of living creatively, in each moment, in a never-ending process of becoming and fully relating. While understanding the nature of reality and doing our best to live with the oppositions, we hold fast to our ideals.

And lately I've come to see that I'm not just a descendant within this tradition, shaped by the stories of those who have gone before me. I'm also an ancestor. I can and do help create the future. I can look to and embody, and represent, the best in Ananda Marga, and bring that energy to whatever undertaking I engage in. I can help to write a new story. I remain optimistic about AM's future and the role it can play on our planet.

Not long ago I met an acharya who traveled the world doing relief work. He was an expert at constructing dome buildings out of renewable materials, and had been invited to advise on rebuilding earthquake-damaged villages in Pakistan. He worked with Muslim builders, with NGO officials, taking moments out of the day to do his sadhana and half-bath (a practice the Muslims appreciated as similar to theirs). He was being the change he wanted to see in the world. No tall talks or boring lectures, just serving his brothers and sisters. This, he said, was what Baba wanted us to do—build a world family.

There are many people like this who inspire me greatly. Mystics and activists, these people are drawn to discover what lies beneath the surface patterns of the world. Edging their way across the earth's shining fields, they take hold of the material of the cosmic tapestry, and with a jerk, lay it straight. It's like yanking a tablecloth out from underneath a full set of china, and then peering down those now-straight lines of consciousness into the origins of the world.

This, I suspect, is what I crossed the planet as a young man to hear: not only do we all spiral out of the mind of God to dance like angels on the heads of protons for a short while. But we spiral back in again, following the threads home.

Baba put it this way: "A child has played outside for the whole day. As evening approaches he thinks that his father must have returned home. 'Let me return home and sit near him,' he thinks. When one is tired of this world and of worldliness, he yearns to go back to spirituality—his home." Beyond the dazzling repetitions, the warp and the weave, beckons the One who rolled all these things into motion.

This is the promise of yoga and of Tantra, a promise that slowly came to fruition within me over the years of living abroad, as I moved from darkness to light in my emotional and spiritual lives. Each day now I try to find a way of living fully in the world while laying claim to its fundamentally transcendent nature, perceiving its essential connectivity.

Bringing heaven down to earth.

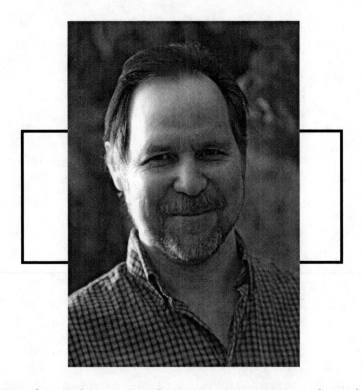

Andy Douglas was born in Brazil to missionary parents, and travel and spiritual practice have shaped his life ever since. He has practiced yoga and meditation for thirty years, and lived for seven years in various countries of Asia, four of those as a monk. After returning to the U. S. from Korea in 1990, he worked as a journalist and public radio announcer, before receiving a bachelors' degree in anthropology from the University of Iowa. In 2005 he received an MFA in Creative Writing, also from the University of Iowa, where he was the recipient of the Marcus Bach Fellowship for Writing about Religion and Culture. He also translates and sings Bengali devotional songs and has created a CD *Into the Mystic: Songs of Prabhat Ranjan Sarkar.* The author is active in peace, economic justice, and prison issues, and sings in a choir with prisoners. He lives in Iowa City.

Bottom Dog Press

Other Titles in Our Memoir Series

The Way-Back Room: A Memoir of a Detroit Childhood
by Mary Minock
218 pgs. $17.00

Hunger Artist: A Suburban Childhood
by Joanne Jacobson130 pgs. $16.00

Second Story Woman: A Memoir of Second Chances
by Carol Calladine
226 pgs. $15.00

*120 Charles Street, The Village: Journals and
Writings 1949-1950*
by Holly Beye
236 pgs. $15.00

Milltown Natural: Essays and Stories from a Life
by Richard Hague
182 (hard cover) $16.00

Milldust and Roses: Memoirs
by Larry Smith
150 pgs. $12.00

Writing Work: Writers on Working-Class Writing
edited by David Shevin, Larry Smith, Janet Zandy
222 pgs. $12.00

Most of the 70 some books of poetry
that we have published also include memoir.

Bottom Dog Press
PO Box 425, Huron, OH 44839
http://smithdocs.net

CPSIA information can be obtained at www.ICGtesting.com
Printed in the USA
LVOW08s0918231113

362532LV00002B/141/P